a guy's guide to great eating

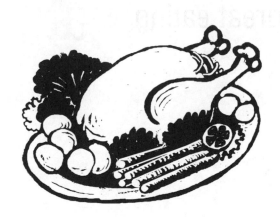

a guy's guide
to great eating

big-flavored, fat-reduced recipes

for men who love to eat

Don Mauer

HOUGHTON MIFFLIN COMPANY
BOSTON   NEW YORK   1999

With love, to my father, DONALD L. MAUER,

who left this earth far too early, but who was the first guy

to show me how much fun cooking could be.

Copyright © 1999 by Don Mauer & Associates, Inc.

For information about permission to reproduce selections from
this book, write to Permissions, Houghton Mifflin Company,
215 Park Avenue South, New York, New York 10003.

Library of Congress Cataloging-in-Publication Data

Mauer, Don.
  A guy's guide to great eating : big-flavored, fat-reduced
recipes for men who love to eat / Don Mauer.
    p.   cm.
Includes index
ISBN 0-395-91536-8
1. Cookery, American. 2. Reducing diets—Recipes.
I. Title.
  TX715.M454   1999
  641.5973—dc21   99-11028   CIP

Book design and drawings by Anne Chalmers
Typefaces: Adobe Caslon, Helvetica Condensed,
Akzidenz Grotesque

Printed in the United States of America

RRD 10 9 8 7 6 5 4 3 2 1

Preface

I wrote this book to share my food and ideas with as many people as possible, especially guys. I love good food and you must too, or you wouldn't be holding this book in your hands. I have always believed great-tasting food can also be healthful. I use the freshest ingredients I can find, with the least amount of fat and oil possible.

Most of my recipes get 25 percent or less of their calories from fat. Why? I believe that is the healthiest balance in a food plan. Keeping the fat of each recipe low also makes it easier to decide what you want to make. You can relax, knowing the calories from fat will almost always be at a healthy level. You can prepare what you want based on your palate, not on your calculator. What sounds good? What gets your heart beating a little faster? The answers to those questions will lead you in the right direction.

As has always been true since I started spreading the word about great-tasting, healthful eating, I'd like you to write to me. If you find sustenance within these covers, write to me. If you have a great-tasting, healthful recipe you'd like to share with me, share it. If you have a favorite recipe that is way too high in fat or calories and you want to make it more healthful, send it to me. If this book touches your life in a positive way, share your thoughts with me at:

P.O. Box 1363
Cary, NC 27512-1363

Or by email at: leanwizard@aol.com

I can hardly wait to hear from you.

Contents

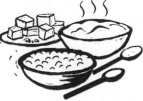

Introduction

I'll admit it: like most men, I love to eat—a lot. When I tried to get my eating habits under control—doctor's orders—the tiny portions made me want to run to the nearest steakhouse for a man-size meal. I reached the end of my rope with a recipe for light macaroni and cheese. The fat level was fine. The calorie count looked good. But the serving size stopped me cold: one-half cup. Come on! I want to meet the man who eats a half cup of macaroni and cheese and can't eat another bite because he's so stuffed. *Puh-leeze.*

A single four-inch buttermilk pancake doesn't fill me up in the morning. A wussy little half sandwich for lunch doesn't keep my furnace fired up all afternoon. And anyone who thinks a three-ounce serving of chicken breast, a half cup of steamed green beans and a small boiled potato will keep me—or most men—from raiding the refrigerator an hour later should think again.

After speaking with hundreds of men and women, I decided to write a cookbook for real guys—not people with the appetite of a supermodel. This book is aimed at both men who cook and the people who cook for men and are concerned about health.

I can't count how many women have approached me and confided, "Last night, I tried a new, low-fat recipe, and my husband barely touched it." These women usually go on to say something like, "If I serve a steak and a baked potato with sour cream and butter, he devours it and asks for more." That's the way I used to eat.

To reduce dinnertime friction, one woman told me that she actually cooks three separate meals: one the kids will eat, one her husband will eat without complaint and one that fits into her healthful diet. Everyone eats what they want, but who wants to be a short-order cook every night?

The recipes in this book should satisfy everybody. The servings are guy-size, but almost every dish gets 25 percent or less of its calories from fat. Every recipe can increase your chances of living a long and healthy life while providing full satisfaction. Each recipe was painstakingly created to satisfy my own tastes.

When I was 15 years old, I taught myself to cook because I loved to eat. Because I loved to eat, I got big—308 pounds. In 1990, I gave my favorite recipes a complete overhaul, trimming fat and slashing calories while creating major flavor. My efforts were so successful that I lost more than 100 pounds and never once felt deprived. My new dishes were so good that a friend told the *Chicago Sun-Times* about me, and before I knew it, I'd gone from running a photo lab to cooking on national television.

Today, I'm 51 years old and in excellent health. Am I slim? Nope. I haven't been slim since I was 9 years old. Am I lean? I'm far leaner than I was in 1989, when I weighed over 300 pounds. Am I as lean as I could be? No. Nonetheless, I've maintained most of my 100-pound weight loss for nearly a decade. I still love to cook, and I still love to eat.

Since I enjoy cooking more than my wife, Susan, does, I'm the head shopper and chef of the household. Because I'm too busy to spend much more than 30 minutes on any meal, my recipes are easy as well as healthful. I have no time to go to a specialty food store for exotic ingredients, and you probably don't either. That's why every ingredient used in this book can be found in most supermarkets.

I've provided complete nutritional information for each recipe, so you can put away your calculator, break out the skillet and get cooking. I've also indicated how much sodium is in every serving, and I've given tips for reducing it throughout the book. If you have a problem with sodium, you can still enjoy almost every recipe.

Most important, these dishes are full of no-holds-barred flavor, so

 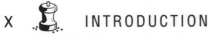

you'll be satisfied from the first bite to the last. In the pages that follow, you'll find real food like buttermilk pancakes and breakfast potatoes, grilled chicken and crunchy Carolina slaw, turkey gumbo and corn bread, meat loaf and whipped potatoes, peppery pork and white beans. You can enjoy crab cakes loaded with crab, succulent sizzling shrimp, spicy oven-fried onion rings, a chicken pot pie better than Mom used to make and a dark chocolate cake with fudgy chocolate frosting. There's a whole section of snacks ready in a flash, including several salsas better than any you can buy at the supermarket.

You'll also find a creamy, cheese-loaded macaroni and cheese that may be the best you've ever tasted, and you can eat a great big belly-filling serving yet remain on a healthful path. That's my kind of eating.

 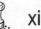

major league
breakfasts

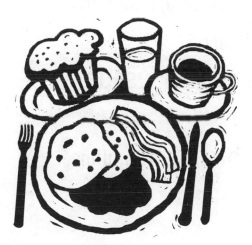

light-as-air buttermilk pancakes

cornmeal blueberry pancakes

sunday morning pecan-topped
french toast casserole

lean scrambled eggs

snappy o'brien breakfast potatoes

oven-roasted bacon

country-style breakfast sausage

apple muffins

pumpkin-raisin breakfast muffins

Breakfast

is a must for me. I don't mean dry toast and half a grapefruit or those diet shakes. If men were meant to drink breakfast, Eve would have handed Adam a can of apple-flavored breakfast drink.

Small breakfasts just aren't enough, especially on the weekend. When I began to lose weight, I learned that my metabolic engine didn't rev up until I ate. If I want to start burning calories, I have to consume some. A tiny breakfast means that I'll need to refuel midmorning, and when I do that, I always seem to eat the wrong thing.

In my old, heavy days, I'd sit down to a butter-drenched pile of pancakes floating in a sea of syrup, a mess of sausages, hash browns, orange juice, coffee with cream and a glass of milk. Unfortunately, breakfasts like those are a prescription for a short life unless you're headed out to the fields for a full day of work.

Today, I still like pancakes for my Sunday breakfast, but now I make them with low-fat buttermilk and drained applesauce, and cook them in a skillet with just a touch of oil. I use a reduced-fat margarine, which has only 15 percent of the fat of butter, and I drizzle on real maple syrup, since it's loaded with flavor and fat-free. I can still enjoy sausage, too, because I created one that's generous with flavor but stingy with fat.

If you're content with a Jerry Seinfeld breakfast of cold cereal and milk, OK. But if you want a hearty breakfast that you'd find at a popular truck stop, without all the fat and calories, read on.

light-as-air buttermilk pancakes

makes 4 five-inch pancakes

In my book, when you're talking pancakes, you're talking buttermilk. It imparts sweet and tangy flavors, but the only butter in it is on the carton label. Buttermilk used to be the thick liquid left over after butter was churned, but today it's made from nonfat or low-fat milk.

3 tablespoons unsweetened applesauce
1 cup all-purpose flour
2 tablespoons granulated sugar (optional)
2 teaspoons baking powder

½ teaspoon salt
1 teaspoon canola oil
1 cup low-fat buttermilk
1 large egg

1. Place a strainer over a bowl deep enough so the bottom of the strainer doesn't touch the bottom of the bowl. Put the applesauce in the strainer and set aside to drain for 15 minutes; you should have 2 tablespoons drained applesauce. Preheat the oven to 170 degrees.

2. Meanwhile, in a medium mixing bowl, stir together the flour, sugar, if using, baking powder and salt until combined. Set aside.

3. Place a medium heavy-bottomed, well-seasoned skillet over medium heat and add the canola oil.

4. While the skillet is heating, put the drained applesauce, buttermilk and egg in a medium mixing bowl and whisk until combined. Add the flour mixture and whisk until almost smooth.

5. Fold a paper towel into eighths and, using it as a pad, spread the canola oil over the surface of the skillet. Place the pad, oil side down, on a saucer near the skillet. When a few drops of water skitter and dance on the surface of the skillet, pour a generous ½ cup of the batter into the center. Tip the skillet gently to spread out the batter a little. Cook until bubbles appear in the center of the pancake, about 2 minutes. Flip the pancake over and cook for 2 minutes more, or until it springs back when pressed in the center. As each pancake is done, transfer it to an ovenproof plate, cover with a couple of paper towels and keep warm in the oven. Continue until the batter is gone and serve.

Nutritional information per pancake: 186 calories (10.5% from fat), 2.2 g fat (0.8 g saturated fat), 6.8 g protein, 31.6 g carbohydrate, 57 mg cholesterol, 365 mg sodium.

saltsense: Omitting the salt reduces the sodium to 99 mg per pancake.

leansuggestions: During blueberry season, make blueberry buttermilk pancakes. Pour the batter for a single pancake into the skillet, then distribute 10 to 12 washed and dried blueberries over the batter. Proceed as directed.

- For buckwheat pancakes, use ½ cup buckwheat flour and ½ cup white flour and proceed as directed.
- For whole wheat pancakes, use ⅓ cup whole wheat flour and ⅔ cup white flour and proceed as directed.
- This recipe may be doubled or tripled, depending on your appetites and the number of guests.

cornmeal blueberry pancakes

makes 16 pancakes

I've loved the flavor of blueberries all my life, and they are at their best in pancakes. The sweet-tasting cornmeal gives these pancakes more body than flour alone would. I serve them with breakfast sausages (page 14) and real maple syrup. A cup of black, fresh-brewed drip coffee is the only other thing I need for a great morning jump-start.

1½ cups fresh blueberries, picked over, washed and drained

¾ cup plus 1½ tablespoons all-purpose flour, *divided*

1 cup yellow cornmeal, preferably stone-ground

1 teaspoon baking powder

½ teaspoon baking soda

¼ teaspoon salt

1 large egg, *separated*

1 tablespoon canola oil, plus more for oiling pan

2 cups low-fat buttermilk

2 tablespoons clover or other mild honey

1. Place the oven rack in the center and preheat the oven to 170 degrees.

2. Stir together the blueberries and 1½ tablespoons of the flour in a small bowl until the blueberries are coated. Set aside.

3. Put the remaining ¾ cup flour, cornmeal, baking powder, baking soda and salt in a large bowl and stir until well combined. Set aside.

4. Add the egg yolk and oil to a 1-quart bowl and whisk until blended. Add the buttermilk and honey, whisking until combined. Set aside.

5. Add the egg white to a separate small bowl and beat with an electric mixer on high until stiff but not dry. Set aside.

6. Form a well in the dry ingredients, add the buttermilk mixture and the blueberries and stir until combined. Gently fold the beaten egg white into the batter.

7. Place a large heavy-bottomed nonstick skillet over medium heat. When a few drops of water skitter and dance on the surface, lightly spray it with vegetable oil. Pour ¼ cup batter into the skillet for each pancake. Cook until the top of each pancake is covered with bubbles and the edges appear dry, about 2 minutes. Flip the pancakes over and cook until the bottoms are golden, 1½ to 2 minutes. As each pancake is done, transfer it to an ovenproof plate, cover with a couple of paper towels and keep warm in the oven. Continue, first spraying the skillet's surface with vegetable oil, until the batter is gone, and serve.

Nutritional information per pancake: 98 calories (21.3% from fat), 2.3 g fat (0.2 g saturated fat), 2.8 g protein, 16.4 g carbohydrate, 13 mg cholesterol, 118 mg sodium.

leansuggestions: Nonfat or low-fat margarine may be used to top each pancake. For a special treat, serve with real maple syrup.

◆ Frozen, thawed blueberries may be substituted for fresh.

sunday morning pecan-topped french toast casserole

makes 6 servings

Originally, this recipe had almost 700 calories per serving. If that wasn't bad enough, each serving packed in almost 44 grams of fat (57.7 percent of calories). Wow! It was one tasty breakfast dish, but it exceeded my fat allowance for an entire day.

The fat came from half-and-half, whole eggs, a stick of butter and a cup of pecans. I made some substitutions, but maintained the rich taste and delightful pecan flavor. Start preparing this dish the day before you plan to serve it.

1 8-ounce French bread, cut into 1-inch-thick slices
1½ cups whole milk
1½ cups evaporated skim milk
6 large egg whites (or ¾ cup nonfat egg substitute)
2 large eggs
1 teaspoon vanilla extract
⅛ teaspoon fresh-grated nutmeg
⅛ teaspoon ground cinnamon

topping
1 cup packed light brown sugar
1 ½-ounce packet Butter Buds, mixed with ½ cup hot water
2 tablespoons dark corn syrup
1 ounce pecans, finely chopped (¼ cup)

1. Lightly spray a 13-by-9-inch baking dish with vegetable oil. Place the bread slices on their sides in the baking dish (crowding is OK). The dish will be completely covered with bread and filled to the top.

2. In a large mixing bowl, whisk together the milk, evaporated milk, egg whites, eggs, vanilla, nutmeg and cinnamon until combined. Pour over the bread slices, cover the dish with foil and refrigerate overnight.

3. **The next morning, make the topping:** In a medium mixing bowl, whisk together the brown sugar, Butter Buds and corn syrup until the sugar dissolves.

4. Preheat the oven to 350 degrees.

5. Drizzle the topping evenly over the bread slices. Sprinkle with the pecans. Bake, uncovered, until puffed and golden, about 40 minutes. Remove from the oven and let stand for 5 minutes before serving.

Nutritional information per serving: 391 calories (18.8% from fat), 8.2 g fat, 16.7 g protein, 63 g carbohydrates, 81 mg cholestcrol, 545 mg sodium.

leansuggestion: This casserole is sweet, so serve it with some lean ham browned in a touch of vegetable oil in a nonstick skillet. Or serve with Oven-Roasted Bacon (page 12).

lean scrambled eggs

makes 2 servings

I learned to make scrambled eggs when I was 10 years old. My brothers and I would get up early on Saturday morning and make breakfast for our folks. As the oldest, I was in charge of the eggs. I don't know how well those breakfasts *really* turned out, but I do remember that my mom and dad ate every bite.

Later, I learned that scrambled eggs taste even better when small pieces of butter are added to the eggs as they cook. I've even made scrambled eggs in a double boiler to see if they could be soft and creamy without being too wet. (They can, but it's a pain.)

Those days are long gone—but not the scrambled eggs. Using just one yolk delivers the expected yellow color, with only three fat grams per serving, while the whites provide a fluffy, nearly fat-free result.

6 large egg whites
1 large egg

Salt and fresh-ground black pepper

1. Put the egg whites into a small bowl. Break the whole egg into the bowl. Season with salt and pepper and whisk until thoroughly combined.

2. Lightly spray a small nonstick skillet with vegetable oil and place over medium heat. When the skillet is hot, pour in the eggs. As soon as they begin to solidify, use a spatula to push them from the edge of the pan to the center, forming curds. Lift the skillet from the heat and tilt from side to side as you push. As the eggs absorb more heat, the curds will form faster. When the curds are soft and no liquid remains in the skillet, transfer the eggs to a plate. Serve immediately.

Nutritional information per serving (without salt): 93 calories (28.7% from fat), 2.9 g fat (0.9 g saturated fat), 15 g protein, 1.2 g carbohydrate, 107 mg cholesterol, 197 mg sodium.

snappy o'brien breakfast potatoes

makes 4 servings

Healthful breakfast potatoes start with cooked potatoes. Uncooked potatoes take too long to fry and drink up fat.

I always bake a couple of extra potatoes whenever I make them for dinner. Then I cool and refrigerate them so they're ready for action in the morning.

2 baked potatoes, chilled
2 teaspoons bacon grease
1 teaspoon olive oil
½ cup fine-chopped onion
½ cup fine-chopped red bell pepper

1 jalapeño pepper, seeds and stem removed, finely chopped
Salt and fresh-ground black pepper

1. Do not peel the potatoes. Cut them into ⅜-inch cubes. Set aside.

2. Place a nonstick skillet over medium-high heat, and when it is hot, add the bacon grease and oil. When the oil shimmers and starts to smoke, add the onion and bell pepper. When they begin to sizzle, add the diced potatoes. Stir the potatoes around so they are in a single layer. Cook for 3 to 4 minutes, then flip the potatoes over, section by section, and cook for 3 to 4 minutes more. Cook, flipping the potatoes occasionally, for 2 minutes more, or until nicely browned. Season with salt and pepper to taste. Serve immediately.

Nutritional information per serving (without salt): 150 calories (21% from fat), 3.5 g fat (0.5 g saturated fat), 3 g protein, 28 g carbohydrate, 0 mg cholesterol, 9 mg sodium.

cooking tip: If you don't have bacon grease, use 1 tablespoon olive oil.

oven-roasted bacon

makes 4 servings, 2 strips each

If I select the leanest bacon I can find (I check through almost every package before I decide) and roast it instead of frying it, I can make it much leaner than it normally is.

Oscar Mayer bacon was the only kind on our table when I was growing up in the Chicago area, and I still believe it has the best taste of any nationally available brand. If I can find it, I also enjoy John Morrell Hardwood Smoked Bacon.

If I still lived in the Chicago area, I would head for a butcher shop on the far North Side called Bornhofen's, at 6155 North Broadway. Bornhofen's has slab bacon with whole allspice pounded into the rind. It's hand-sliced while you wait. Now that's good bacon.

Do I have bacon with my breakfast every day? No. But once a month, on a Sunday, I roast some and enjoy the heck out of it.

8 ounces thick-sliced bacon, the leaner the better

1. Place the oven rack in the top position and preheat the oven to 425 degrees.

2. Line a jelly-roll pan with aluminum foil. Select a wire rack that fits comfortably inside the pan. Lay the bacon strips side by side on the rack, edges just touching. Bake for 10 minutes. Turn the bacon over and bake for 10 minutes more, or until golden brown. Drain the bacon on several layers of paper towels and serve.

Nutritional information per 2 strips: 91 calories (77% from fat), 7.8 g fat (2.7 g saturated fat), 4.8 g protein, trace of carbohydrate, 13.5 mg cholesterol, 253 mg sodium.

leantip: Trimming some of the fat off the bacon before or after roasting can make a substantial difference.

leansuggestions: Roast more bacon than you need for breakfast and refrigerate what you don't eat. Then, when you want to make Classic Clubhouse Sandwich (page 256), you'll save yourself a step.

- ◆ Save ¼ cup of the bacon grease, refrigerated, for future sautéing. I qualify this recommendation by suggesting that you use no more than 2 teaspoons of bacon grease per dish. This small amount adds only 9 fat grams to the entire dish, but the flavor is well worth the 2 or 3 fat grams per serving.

country-style breakfast sausage

makes 16 patties

For me, a weekend breakfast just isn't breakfast without a couple of sausage patties. The lower-fat patties available at the supermarket aren't very low in fat, so I make my own.

Sage gives this sausage its distinctive flavor. A strong punch of black pepper and cayenne pepper lifts it out of the ordinary.

2 pounds pork tenderloin, trimmed of all visible fat and cut into 1½-inch cubes

1 large garlic clove, mashed to a paste with 2 teaspoons kosher or sea salt

2 teaspoons minced fresh sage leaves or 1 teaspoon dry rubbed sage

1½ teaspoons fresh-ground black pepper

¼ teaspoon cayenne pepper
Pinch of fresh-grated nutmeg

1. Lightly spray a jelly-roll pan with vegetable oil. Place the pork cubes in the pan in a single layer and put the pan in the freezer, uncovered, for 45 minutes, or until the meat is partially frozen.

2. Place one-quarter of the pork in a food processor with the steel blade in place and process, pulsing, until coarsely ground and crumbly—no more than 15 pulses. (The pork may also be run twice through an electric or hand-cranked meat grinder, using the coarse plate.)

3. In a large mixing bowl, combine the garlic-salt paste, sage, black pepper, cayenne pepper and nutmeg. Add the ground pork and, using clean hands or a rubber spatula, combine thoroughly with the seasonings. Chill in the refrigerator for 1 hour to allow the flavors to blend.

4. Form the pork mixture into sixteen 2-ounce patties. (At this point, the patties may be frozen for future use.) Place a large sauté pan over medium heat and lightly spray with vegetable oil. Place half the patties in the pan and cook for 4 minutes per side, or until they are no longer pink in the center and offer resistance when pressed. Continue with the remaining patties. Serve.

Nutritional information per 2-ounce patty: 69 calories (25.4% from fat), 1.9 g fat (0.7 g saturated fat), 11.9 g protein, 0.3 g carbohydrate, 37 mg cholesterol, 162 mg sodium.

cookingtip: Turning garlic into paste is easy. Smash the garlic clove with the side of a knife; remove and discard the skin. Press the garlic through a garlic press onto a clean cutting board. Spread the garlic out flat with the side of the knife, sprinkle with the salt and drag the side of the knife over the garlic several times, using strong downward pressure.

apple muffins

makes 15 muffins

I've always liked a good muffin, and when I weighed more than 300 pounds, I often picked up a couple on my way to work. The paper bag the muffins came in would have grease stains on it by the time I arrived at my desk. Should have been a clue, right?

Now, I'll stir these muffins together on Saturday afternoon. Then I can take them to work during the week and enjoy them, knowing they are low in fat.

By the way, these muffins can be made with blueberries, peaches, strawberries or cherries, substituted measure for measure for the apples.

3 tablespoons unsweetened applesauce
2 medium Granny Smith apples, peeled, cored and diced into ¼-inch pieces (about 2 cups)
1½ cups all-purpose flour, *divided*
2 teaspoons baking powder
½ teaspoon baking soda
½ teaspoon ground cinnamon

¼ teaspoon salt
1 large egg yolk
2 tablespoons canola oil
½ cup low-fat buttermilk
3 large egg whites
1 teaspoon vanilla extract
¾ cup granulated sugar

1. Place a strainer over a bowl deep enough so the bottom of the strainer doesn't touch the bottom of the bowl. Put the applesauce in the strainer and set aside to drain for 15 minutes; you should have 2 tablespoons drained applesauce.

2. Meanwhile, place the oven rack in the center and preheat the oven to 375 degrees. Put foil muffin liners into 15 muffin cups and spray lightly with butter-flavored vegetable oil. Set aside.

3. Put the apples and ½ cup of the flour into a medium mixing bowl and stir until the apples are coated with the flour. Set aside.

4. Put the remaining 1 cup flour, baking powder, baking soda, cinnamon and salt in a medium mixing bowl and stir until combined. Set aside.

5. Put the egg yolk and oil into a large mixing bowl. Whisk until combined. Add the buttermilk, egg whites, drained applesauce and vanilla and whisk until combined. Add the sugar and whisk until dissolved. Stir in the apples. Add the flour mixture and stir until just moistened.

6. Spoon the batter into the prepared muffin cups, filling each about two-thirds full. Bake until the muffins are golden brown and a toothpick inserted into the center of a muffin comes out clean, 25 to 28 minutes. Cool in the pan on a rack. Serve warm or at room temperature.

Nutritional information per muffin: 122 calories (18% from fat), 2.4 g fat (0.3 g saturated fat), 2.4 g protein, 23 g carbohydrate, 14.2 mg cholesterol, 132 mg sodium.

lean suggestions: Once they have cooled, keep the muffins covered and refrigerated.
- To keep the diced apples from turning brown before baking, sprinkle them with lemon juice and drain just before adding them.
- These muffins keep well frozen and may be reheated in a 300-degree oven for 10 minutes.
- They are terrific served warm with Never-Better Roasted Pork Loin (page 86).
- They are also great as a snack, warmed in a microwave oven (12 to 15 seconds on high) and smeared with low-fat or nonfat cream cheese.

pumpkin-raisin breakfast muffins

makes 24 muffins

The seasonings in these muffins remind me of pumpkin pie, and the tops rise high out of the pan. Don't worry about the butter. You may not believe it by the taste, but the muffins *are* low in fat.

Pumpkin is loaded with beta-carotene and fiber. The raisins contain iron and more fiber. It's hard to think of these as healthful, since they taste so darn good.

¾ cup unsweetened applesauce
3½ cups all-purpose flour
2 teaspoons baking soda
1 teaspoon salt
1 teaspoon ground cinnamon
1 teaspoon fresh-grated nutmeg

½ cup unsalted butter, at room temperature
3 cups granulated sugar
2 cups canned pumpkin
1 large egg
3 large egg whites
1½ cups raisins

1. Place a strainer over a bowl deep enough so the bottom of the strainer doesn't touch the bottom of the bowl. Put the applesauce in the strainer and set aside to drain for 15 minutes; you should have ½ cup drained applesauce.

2. Meanwhile, place the oven rack in the center and preheat the oven to 375 degrees. Spray two 12-cup muffin pans with a flour-and-vegetable-oil spray, such as Baker's Joy. Set aside.

3. Put the flour, baking soda, salt, cinnamon and nutmeg in a large mixing bowl and stir until combined. Set aside.

4. Put the butter in another large mixing bowl and mix with an electric mixer on medium-high for 3 minutes, or until light.

5. Add the sugar to the batter and mix, scraping down the sides of the bowl from time to time, for 4 minutes, or until light and fluffy.

6. Add the applesauce and pumpkin, and mix for 3 minutes. While the mixer is running, add the egg and mix for 30 seconds, then add each of the egg whites, one at a time, mixing for 30 seconds after each addition.

7. Add the flour mixture, and mix on low until combined. Add the raisins and stir until combined.

8. Spoon the batter into the prepared muffin cups, filling each almost to the top. Place the muffin pans side by side in the oven and bake for 25 to 30 minutes, or until a toothpick inserted into the center of a muffin comes out clean. Cool in the pans on a rack for 5 minutes. Remove the muffins from the pans and let them cool completely on the rack.

Nutritional information per muffin: 235 calories (16.8% from fat), 4.4 g fat (2.5 g saturated fat), 3 g protein, 48.1 g carbohydrate, 19 mg cholesterol, 170 mg sodium.

cookingtip: These muffins keep best when covered and refrigerated. Placed in recloseable freezer bags, they will keep frozen for 6 to 8 weeks.

whopping
good soups

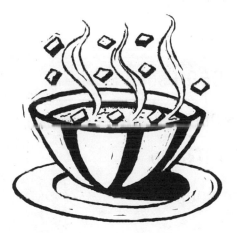

chicken, sausage and corn chowder

southwestern corn and
shrimp chowder

great gawd almighty gumbo

hungarian-style hamburger soup

chill-chasin' split pea soup

hearty lean lentil stew

easy tex-mex pinto bean soup

as good as it gets onion soup

mess o' mushroom soup

effortless tomato soup

cup'a-cup'a soup

I hate sitting down to a bowl of watery broth with tiny pieces of vegetables and microscopic bits of meat. I want huge flavor and big chunks of vegetables and meat—and lots of them. Why make soup if it isn't going to be better than what you get in a can?

My Great Gawd Almighty Gumbo is forcefully seasoned and jam-packed with turkey, green peppers, onions, tomatoes, celery and jalapeño peppers. Chicken, Sausage and Corn Chowder has quick-cooking lentils and smoky low-fat sausage for extra heft and relies on nonfat sour cream instead of the usual high-fat whipping cream.

The foundation of any great soup is the broth. The better it is, the bigger the flavor will be. For that reason, I never use bouillon cubes, which are mostly salt. Some canned broths are decent, but if you have a weekend afternoon available, make your own. It will give you absolute control over the result and is soulfully satisfying.

If you're preparing chicken broth—the basis of most of the soups that follow—you can use bones and skin saved in the freezer from roast chicken dinners. Or head for a natural food store and see if it has backs and necks from naturally raised chickens. These are usually cheap. If backs and necks aren't available, buy legs and thighs, which are less expensive than wings. Broil them until brown and drop them into the pot.

I used to simmer my stockpot on the stove all day on Sunday. Then I created an easier method. After bringing the pot to a simmer, I set the oven temperature to 325 degrees, put the covered pot in the oven and leave it there for six hours while my wife and I go out. Upon our return, the house smells phenomenal and the broth is beautifully golden. Now I always make broth this way. Having homemade broth at hand means you too can make a soup with big-time flavor in short order.

chicken, sausage and corn chowder

makes 6 servings, each 1½ cups

This colorful and delicious soup is high in protein and fiber while delivering only 4 grams of fat per serving. Part of the secret is low-fat sausage, which tastes almost exactly like the high-fat kind. I should tell you up front that this soup takes a bit of work. There's some slicing and dicing before it hits the bowl. BUT—and that's a big but—it's absolutely fabulous.

1 tablespoon olive oil

7 ounces low-fat kielbasa sausage, split lengthwise and cut into ¼-inch-thick slices

¾ cup chopped onion

3 cups fat-free reduced-sodium chicken broth, *divided*

1½ cups frozen corn kernels

1 baking (russet) potato (about 8 ounces), peeled and cut into ½-inch dice

1 cooked skinless, boneless chicken breast half, cut into bite-size pieces

(about 1 cup)

½ cup lentils, picked over and rinsed

1 bay leaf

1 cup nonfat sour cream

1 cup packed fresh spinach leaves, washed and thinly sliced

½ teaspoon salt

½ teaspoon fresh-ground black pepper

1 tablespoon chopped fresh parsley leaves

1. Place a 4-quart heavy-bottomed saucepan over medium-high heat and add the oil. When the oil is hot, add the kielbasa and cook, stirring, until lightly browned, about 4 minutes. Using a slotted spoon, transfer the kielbasa to a double layer of paper towels. Set aside.

2. Add the onion to the pan and cook, stirring frequently, until golden, 6 to 7 minutes. Add ½ cup of the broth and simmer for 2 minutes, scraping up the browned bits. Add the remaining 2½ cups broth, kielbasa, corn, potato, chicken, lentils and bay leaf. Reduce the heat to medium and simmer, covered, for 25 minutes, or until the potato and lentils are tender.

3. Whisk the sour cream into the soup. Stir in the spinach, salt and pepper, reduce the heat to low and cook until the soup is just heated through and the spinach is wilted, 2 to 3 minutes. (Do not let it boil.) Remove the bay leaf and serve immediately, sprinkled with the parsley.

Nutritional information per serving: 250 calories (14.7% from fat), 4.1 g fat (0.9 g saturated fat), 19.8 g protein, 35.6 g carbohydrate, 15 mg cholesterol, 709 mg sodium.

leansuggestions: Substitute Homemade Jimdandy Kielbasa Sausage (page 82) for store-bought kielbasa. Break up with a spoon and proceed as directed.

♦ Bruce Aidells produces some of the best-tasting sausages anywhere. Aidells sausage is available in many large supermarkets. Look for one that is lower in fat and substitute it for the kielbasa.

saltsense: Using no-salt-added chicken broth and omitting the ½ teaspoon salt will reduce the sodium by more than half—to 333 mg per serving.

 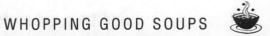

southwestern corn and shrimp chowder

makes 4 servings, each 1⅔ cups

I would pay top dollar for a bowl of this soup in any good restaurant. The jalapeño pepper and salsa provide just enough heat to enhance all the flavors. A squeeze of lime juice at the end is magical. Taste the chowder before adding the juice to see what I mean.

1 tablespoon butter
1 small onion, chopped (about ¾ cup)
1½ cups corn kernels (fresh, if possible)
1 tablespoon clover or other mild honey
2½ cups fat-free reduced-sodium chicken broth
¼ cup prepared tomato salsa (I use Newman's Own, medium-hot)
1 pound medium shrimp, cooked, shelled, deveined and coarsely chopped
½ cup nonfat sour cream

¼ cup fine-chopped fresh cilantro
2 tablespoons fine-chopped fresh basil leaves
1 jalapeño pepper, seeded and minced (if you like some heat, leave the seeds)
½ teaspoon salt
¼ teaspoon fresh-ground black pepper, or to taste
Lime wedges

1. Place a 4-quart saucepan over medium heat and add the butter. When it begins to foam, add the onion and cook, stirring occasionally, until softened, about 6 minutes. Add the corn and honey and cook, stirring occasionally, for 3 minutes.

2. Add the broth and simmer, stirring occasionally, for 5 minutes, or until the corn is just tender. Add the salsa and simmer, covered, for 5 minutes. Add the shrimp, sour cream, cilantro, basil, jalapeño, salt and pepper, and cook, uncovered, until just heated through (do not let it boil). Taste and adjust the seasonings. Serve immediately with the lime wedges on the side.

a guy's guide to great eating

Nutritional information per serving: 268 calories (19.1% from fat), 5.7 9 g fat (2.3 g saturated fat), 29.2 g protein, 26 g carbohydrate, 186 mg cholesterol, 568 mg sodium.

leansuggestion: You can substitute 1 pound of uncooked bay scallops for the shrimp.

saltsense: Substituting no-salt-added chicken broth reduces the sodium to 320 mg per serving.

great gawd almighty gumbo

makes 6 servings, each 1½ cups

My lean version of gumbo is the solution to all those Thanksgiving leftovers, but it tastes so sensational, you won't want to save it for the big bird. My gumbo can easily be made at any time of the year with chicken breasts.

The gumbo filé powder used in this recipe is actually ground sassafras leaves. In the South, it's available at every grocery store. If you can't find it where you live, contact Penzeys Spices at (414) 679-7207. If you want to make gumbo without the filé powder, that's OK, too; as far as I know, there is no substitute for it.

1 tablespoon olive oil	8 ounces cooked turkey or chicken breast, diced
1 medium onion, diced	1¼ cups long-grain white rice
1 medium green bell pepper, chopped	1 bay leaf
1 medium tomato, peeled, seeded and chopped	½ teaspoon dried oregano, crumbled
1 cup sliced fresh okra	½ teaspoon onion powder
2 celery ribs, strings removed, chopped	¼ teaspoon dried thyme, crumbled
4 scallions, chopped	¼ teaspoon dried basil, crumbled
½ jalapeño pepper, minced	½ teaspoon salt
2 large garlic cloves, chopped	½ teaspoon fresh-ground black pepper
4 tablespoons all-purpose flour	1½ teaspoons filé powder
6 cups turkey broth, skimmed of all fat (fat-free reduced-sodium chicken broth may be substituted)	

1.   Place a 5-quart saucepan over medium heat and add the oil. When the oil is hot, add the onion, bell pepper, tomato, okra, celery, scallions, jalapeño and garlic. Sauté until the onion is tender and translucent, about 5 minutes. Add the flour and cook, stirring, for several minutes. (The flour will stick to the bottom of the saucepan; don't be concerned.)

2.   Add the broth to the pan, stirring to break up any flour lumps and scraping up the flour from the bottom of the pan. Stir in the turkey or chicken, rice, bay leaf, oregano, onion powder, thyme, basil, salt and pepper. Reduce the heat to low and gently simmer for 30 minutes.

3.   Remove the pan from the heat and remove the bay leaf. Whisk in the filé powder. Taste and adjust the seasonings. Serve immediately.

Nutritional information per serving (using chicken broth): 268 calories (9.7% from fat), 2.9 g fat (0.4 g saturated fat), 17 g protein, 42.7 g carbohydrate, 31 mg cholesterol, 629 mg sodium.

leansuggestion: If fresh okra is not available, substitute frozen. Add it with the broth in step 2.

cookingtip: It's best not to let the soup return to a boil once you add the filé powder, because the texture can become gummy. If you are refrigerating the soup to serve later, whisk in the filé powder at serving time, after heating the gumbo through.

saltsense: Omitting the salt and using no-salt-added chicken broth or homemade no-salt-added turkey broth reduces the sodium by more than two-thirds.

hungarian-style hamburger soup

makes 6 servings, each 1½ cups

When I was a kid, Grandmother Mauer made a fresh hamburger soup. It took me a long time to duplicate it, but I finally created a version I like. I use the leanest ground beef I can find and increase the amount of onions again and again, since I like their sweet flavor against the heartiness of the beef. This soup is very close to my grandmother's. The best thing about it is that it's so quick to cook. In 50 minutes it's on the table, and it brings less than 6 fat grams with it.

2 teaspoons olive oil
3 medium onions, coarsely chopped
1 pound 93% lean ground beef
3 tablespoons all-purpose flour
2 teaspoons paprika (I prefer imported Hungarian paprika)
½ teaspoon caraway seeds
½ teaspoon fresh-ground black pepper
Pinch of dried marjoram, crumbled

3 14.5-ounce cans beef broth, skimmed of all fat
1½ tablespoons cider vinegar
3 medium red-skin or white potatoes, cut into ½-inch cubes
3 tablespoons chopped fresh parsley

1. Place a heavy-bottomed 5-quart saucepan over medium heat and add the oil. When it is hot, add the onions and cook, stirring, until soft, 5 to 6 minutes. Add the ground beef and cook, breaking it up with a spoon, until it loses its pink color, about 5 minutes. Pour off the liquid and fat, add the flour and cook, stirring, until golden, about 4 minutes. (The flour will stick to the bottom of the saucepan; don't be concerned.) Add the paprika, caraway seeds, pepper and marjoram and stir until fragrant.

 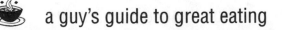

Stir in the broth, vinegar and ¼ cup water, scraping up the flour from the bottom of the pan. Reduce the heat to medium-low and simmer, covered, for 15 minutes.

2.   Add the potatoes to the soup and simmer, covered, for 20 minutes more, or until a potato cube can be easily pierced with the point of a knife. Serve immediately, sprinkled with the parsley.

Nutritional information per serving: 209 calories (24.2% from fat), 5.6 g fat (1.7 g saturated fat), 19.7 g protein, 20.8 g carbohydrate, 46 mg cholesterol, 802 mg sodium.

saltsense: I've added no salt to this soup, because 95 percent of the sodium comes from the canned broth. If you are on a sodium-restricted food plan, substitute no-salt-added beef broth. Alternatively, use your own homemade no-salt-added beef broth.

 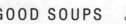

chill-chasin' split pea soup

makes 8 servings, each 1½ cups

Nothing tastes better and warms you to the bottom of your feet more than split pea soup. This soup has a big, hearty flavor, thanks to the slab bacon. Trimming off the visible bacon fat and skimming the soup at the end helps to keep the fat and calorie count at reasonable levels without cutting into the taste.

6 ounces very lean smoked slab bacon	12 ounces (about 1¾ cups) green split peas
1 teaspoon olive oil	8 ounces red-skin or white potatoes, peeled and diced
1½ cups chopped onions	
2 celery ribs, strings removed, chopped	1 bay leaf
2 garlic cloves, crushed	½ teaspoon fresh-ground black pepper
8 cups fat-free reduced-sodium chicken broth	

1. Trim as much of the fat from the bacon as possible and discard. Place a 5-quart saucepan over medium heat and add the oil. When the oil is hot, add the bacon and cook until it just starts to brown around the edges, about 6 minutes. Add the onions and celery and cook, stirring occasionally, until transparent, 5 to 6 minutes. Add the garlic and cook for 2 minutes, or until soft, taking care not to brown it. Add the broth, split peas, potatoes and bay leaf and bring to a boil. Reduce the heat to low and simmer for 1½ hours, or until the peas are very tender.

2. Carefully skim any fat from the soup's surface. Remove the bay leaf. Season with pepper and serve immediately.

 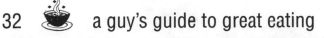

Nutritional information per serving: 172 calories (9.6% from fat), 1.9 g fat (0.4 g saturated fat), 13 g protein, 27.7 g carbohydrate, 7 mg cholesterol, 698 mg sodium.

cooking**tip**: You can substitute thick-sliced bacon for slab bacon.

saltsense: Using no-salt-added chicken broth reduces the sodium to 301 mg per serving.

hearty lean lentil stew

makes 4 servings

Lentils are one of the best beans around. They cook in less than 25 minutes and need no soaking. Originally, this stew relied on bacon for flavor, but bacon, no matter how it is prepared, is loaded with fat. I went with a lean, center-cut smoked pork chop. The pork chops adds good, smoky depth to the stew, and lemon peel brightens the flavors.

1 4-ounce smoked center-cut pork chop, trimmed of all visible fat
1 tablespoon olive oil
1 medium onion, finely diced
2 leeks, white part only, trimmed, washed and finely diced
2 medium carrots, peeled and finely diced
2 celery ribs, strings removed, finely diced
1 large garlic clove, minced
3 tablespoons tomato paste
3 cups fat-free reduced-sodium chicken broth
1 cup lentils, picked over and rinsed

1 thin strip lemon peel
1 bay leaf
½ teaspoon dried thyme leaves, crumbled
Pinch of caraway seeds
1 tablespoon cider vinegar
½ teaspoon salt
½ teaspoon fresh-ground black pepper
1 tablespoon minced fresh parsley leaves

1. Cut the meat from the pork bone and chop it finely. Place a 5-quart saucepan over medium-high heat and add the oil. When the oil is hot, add the chopped pork and the bone. Cook, stirring, until the meat and bone begin to brown slightly, about 4 minutes.

 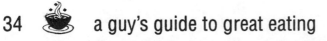

2. Add the onion, leeks, carrots, celery and garlic to the saucepan and cook, stirring frequently, until softened, about 7 minutes. Add the tomato paste and stir until evenly distributed. Add the broth, lentils, lemon peel, bay leaf, thyme and caraway seeds and bring to a boil. Reduce the heat to low and simmer, covered, stirring occasionally, for 30 minutes, or until the lentils are tender.

3. Remove the pork bone, lemon peel and bay leaf. Stir in the vinegar, salt and pepper. Serve immediately, sprinkling each serving with the parsley.

Nutritional information per serving: 285 calories (18% from fat), 5.7 g fat (1.1 g saturated fat), 20.5 g protein, 39.6 g carbohydrate, 18 mg cholesterol, 413 mg sodium.

easy tex-mex pinto bean soup

makes 8 servings, each 1½ cups

When I started out in the kitchen, I began with soup because it seemed easy. Starting from scratch with bones, fresh vegetables and meats was time-consuming. After learning the basics, I turned to simpler and faster methods. This soup takes less than an hour to cook, yet its flavors belie the ease of its preparation.

1 tablespoon olive oil
1 large onion, finely chopped
3 garlic cloves, minced
1 red bell pepper, chopped
1½ teaspoons chili powder
1 teaspoon ground cumin
4 cups fat-free reduced-sodium chicken broth, *divided*
1 16-ounce can pureed tomatoes

7 ounces low-fat kielbasa or smoked sausage, cut into ¼-inch-thick slices
¼ cup mild enchilada sauce (not salsa)
2 15-ounce cans pinto beans, drained and rinsed
1½ tablespoons fresh lime juice
⅓ cup chopped fresh cilantro leaves

1. Place a 5-quart saucepan over medium-high heat and add the oil. When the oil is hot, add the onion and garlic and cook, stirring frequently, until golden, 5 to 7 minutes. Add the bell pepper, reduce the heat to medium, cover and cook until softened, 4 to 5 minutes. Add the chili powder and cumin and cook, stirring, for 30 seconds, until fragrant. Add 3 cups of the broth and bring to a boil. Reduce the heat to low, cover and simmer for 20 minutes.

 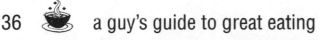

2.   Add the tomatoes, kielbasa or smoked sausage, the remaining 1 cup broth and enchilada sauce, cover partially and simmer, stirring occasionally, for 25 minutes. Add the pinto beans and simmer for 5 minutes more, until heated through. Stir in the lime juice and cilantro and serve.

Nutritional information per serving: 177 calories (15.2% from fat), 2.9 g fat (0.5 g saturated fat), 11.1 g protein, 26 g carbohydrate, 0 mg cholesterol, 649 mg sodium.

saltsense: Using no-salt-added chicken broth and no-salt-added tomatoes reduces the sodium in this soup to 243 mg per serving.

as good as it gets onion soup

makes 8 servings, each 1½ cups

A couple of years ago, a guy wrote to tell me how much he loved the French onion soup in restaurants. He wanted to recreate it at home, but every recipe he found was loaded with butter and cheese.

I knew just what he meant. So, using a recipe of Irena Chalmers's in *The Great Food Almanac* (1994) as the base, I removed most of the fat by substituting olive oil for some of the butter. Then I replaced the high-fat Gruyère cheese with lower-fat mozzarella. Voilà: a healthful, restaurant-quality soup.

1 tablespoon olive oil
1 tablespoon butter
8 medium onions, sliced (about 8 cups)
8 cups reduced-sodium beef broth, skimmed of all fat
½ cup dry red wine
   Fresh-ground black pepper to taste

1 12-ounce loaf French bread, cut into twenty-four ½-inch-thick slices
1½ cups grated part-skim mozzarella cheese

1. Place a large saucepan over medium-high heat and add the oil and butter. Add the onions and stir well to coat. Reduce the heat to low and cook until the onions are soft, about 30 minutes, stirring occasionally. Increase the heat to high and cook about 5 minutes more to brown the onions, stirring constantly. Add the broth and red wine, and season with pepper to taste. Bring to a boil, reduce the heat to low, cover and simmer gently for 30 minutes.

2. Meanwhile, lightly toast the bread slices. When the soup has finished cooking, preheat the broiler.

 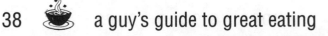

3. Pour the soup into 6 individual broilerproof bowls. Float 4 toasted bread slices on each bowl of soup and top with the grated cheese. Broil until the cheese is melted and lightly browned. Serve immediately.

Nutritional information per serving: 280 calories (29% from fat), 9.2 g fat (4.3 g saturated fat), 13.5 g protein, 34 g carbohydrate, 25 mg cholesterol, 1,229 mg sodium.

saltsense: The high amount of sodium comes from the canned broth and the cheese. Using no-salt-added beef broth reduces the sodium to 409 mg per serving.

mess o' mushroom soup

makes 6 servings, each 1¼ cups

I've always wondered why canned cream of mushroom soups have only a couple of little bits of mushroom in them. When I make my own, I use lots of mushrooms. The original used whipping cream, which, along with the sherry, made my soup very smooth. But almost 200 fat grams glided easily off my guests' spoons. By substituting nonfat sour cream, I created a more healthful version that tastes just as good.

1 tablespoon olive oil	1 teaspoon salt
1 pound white button mushrooms, cleaned and chopped	1½ cups nonfat sour cream, at room temperature
¼ teaspoon cayenne pepper	2 tablespoons all-purpose flour
Pinch of fresh-grated nutmeg	2 tablespoons dry sherry or cognac
4 cups fat-free reduced-sodium chicken broth, *divided*	2 tablespoons chopped fresh parley

1. Place a heavy-bottomed, nonaluminum 4-quart saucepan over medium heat and add the oil. When it is hot, add the mushrooms and sauté for 3 minutes, until they begin to give off liquid. Add the cayenne pepper and nutmeg and sauté for 30 seconds, or until fragrant. Stir in 3 cups of the broth and the salt. Bring to a boil, reduce the heat to medium-low and simmer, uncovered, for 30 minutes, stirring occasionally.

2. Meanwhile, place the sour cream, the remaining 1 cup broth and flour in a medium mixing bowl. Whisk until combined. Set aside.

3. Whisk the sherry or cognac into the soup. Whisk in the sour cream mixture. Imme-

 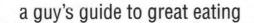

diately reduce the heat to low and cook until just heated through. (Do not let it boil.) Remove from the heat. Ladle the soup into bowls and garnish with the parsley. Serve immediately.

Nutritional information per serving: 140 calories (16.6% from fat), 2.6 g fat (0.3 g saturated fat), 5.5 g protein, 19.4 g carbohydrate, 8 mg cholesterol, 674 mg sodium.

cookingtip: If the soup is too thick, thin it with additional chicken broth.

leansuggestion: Garlic and mushrooms were made for each other. Remove half the cloves from a head of roasted garlic (which can be roasted days ahead and refrigerated; see page 192). In a blender or food processor, puree the garlic with 1 cup of the broth. Add in step 1 and proceed as directed.

saltsense: Omitting the salt will bring the sodium down to 320 mg per serving. Eighty-two percent of the remaining salt comes from the reduced-sodium chicken broth. A significant dent may be made in that 320 mg if no-salt-added chicken broth is used.

effortless tomato soup

makes 6 servings, each 1¼ cups

When I was a kid, lunchtime often meant a cup of canned cream of tomato soup and an egg salad sandwich. Much later, when I was on my own and cooking for myself, I started to make cream of tomato soup from scratch. My soup was better than anything that came from a can: creamy and smooth and loaded with 180 fat grams. I took a few nips and tucks in the original and substituted nonfat sour cream for the whipping cream.

2 teaspoons olive oil	1½ cups nonfat sour cream, at room temperature
1 small onion, minced	
¼ teaspoon cayenne pepper	¼ teaspoon baking soda
Pinch of ground cloves	½ teaspoon clover or other mild honey
1 28-ounce can plum tomatoes	
2 cups fat-free reduced-sodium chicken broth, *divided*	¼ cup sliced fresh basil leaves

1. Place a heavy-bottomed, nonaluminum 4-quart saucepan over medium heat and add the oil. When it is hot, add the onion and sauté for 3 minutes, until softened. Add the cayenne pepper and cloves and sauté for 30 seconds, or until fragrant. Stir in the tomatoes and 1 cup of the chicken broth. Bring to a boil, reduce the heat and simmer, uncovered, for 30 minutes, stirring occasionally and breaking up the tomatoes with the edge of a spoon.

2. Place a strainer over a bowl and strain the soup into the bowl, pressing the solids with the back of a spoon. Return the strained mixture to the saucepan and bring to a simmer over medium-low heat.

 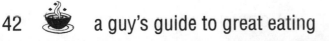

3.   Meanwhile, put the sour cream and the remaining 1 cup chicken broth in a medium mixing bowl. Whisk until combined. Set aside.

4.   When the soup returns to a simmer, stir in the baking soda. (It will foam a little.) Stir in the honey. Add the sour cream mixture and whisk to combine. Cook until just heated through. (Do not let it boil.) Remove from the heat. Taste and adjust the seasonings. Ladle the soup into serving bowls and garnish with the basil. Serve immediately.

Nutritional information per serving: 125 calories (11% from fat), 1.5 g fat (0.2 g saturated fat), 6.2 g protein, 21.7 g carbohydrate, 8 mg cholesterol, 702 mg sodium.

cooking**tip**: If the soup is too thick, thin it with additional chicken broth.

saltsense: A single serving of this soup has 702 mg of sodium. Two-thirds of that comes from the canned tomatoes. Using no-salt-added canned tomatoes salt brings the sodium per serving to a reasonable 218 mg.

cup'a-cup'a soup

makes 10 servings, each 1½ cups

One evening, while I was rushing to come up with a quick dinner, I found two quarts of homemade broth in the back of my refrigerator. I added carrots, green beans, baby peas and yellow corn, along with other vegetables I had on hand, one cup at a time. This soup was the delicious result. It's hearty and flavorful and very close to being fat-free.

8 cups fat-free reduced-sodium chicken broth (or homemade turkey broth, skimmed of all fat)
1 cup diced carrot (about 2 medium)
1 cup raw long-grain white rice
1 cup diced celery (about 2 ribs)
1 cup diced green beans
1 cup frozen baby peas
1 cup frozen corn kernels

1 cup diced ripe tomato (1 medium)
1 cup diced fresh (or frozen) okra (optional)
1½ teaspoons salt (if using canned broth, reduce or omit)
¼ teaspoon fresh-ground black pepper
1 tablespoon cornstarch

1. Bring the broth to a simmer in a 5-quart pot over medium-high heat. Add the carrot and rice. Return to a simmer, reduce the heat to low, cover and simmer for 10 minutes. Add the celery, green beans, peas, corn, tomato, okra (if using), salt (if using) and pepper and simmer for 10 minutes more, or until the rice is cooked.

2. Whisk together ¼ cup water and the cornstarch and then whisk the mixture into the soup. Return the soup to a simmer and allow to thicken slightly. Taste and adjust the seasonings and serve.

 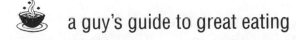

Nutritional information per serving: 123 calories (3.3% from fat), 0.5 g fat (trace of saturated fat), 4.9 g protein, 26.3 g carbohydrate, 0 mg cholesterol, 357 mg sodium.

leansuggestions: Adding 1 cup of diced, cooked chicken breast just before the cornstarch mixture makes this soup even better.

◆   A few shots of Tabasco sauce boost the flavor.

real
meals

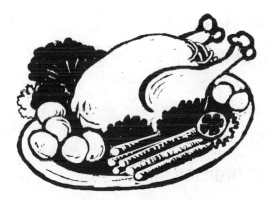

BEEF

a guy's better burger

rubbed and grilled flank steak

cheddar cheeseburger meat loaf

ground beef tortilla roll-ups

slow-cooked pot roast with gravy

kickass beef-chunk chili

billy's chili

lightnin'-fast beefsteak stew

spicy beef and broccoli stir-fry

lean beef goulash

quick hamburger stroganoff

all-beef italian sausage

red peppers stuffed with sausage and rice

baked potatoes with meat sauce

PORK

homemade jimdandy kielbasa sausage

pork chops baked in sour cream

never-better roasted pork loin

southwestern peppery pork with white beans

pork tenderloin with mushrooms and carrots

garlic-and-ginger-flavored grilled pork tenderloin

sweet n' hot onion marmalade

POULTRY

e-z buttermilk-marinated roasted chicken breasts

thai grilled chicken breasts

east indian tandoori chicken breasts

extra-crunchy country-style oven-fried chicken

chicken with olives and peppers

chicken vesuvio

sizzlin' szechuan chicken

succulent sunday supper roast chicken

fat-free sour cream chicken giblet gravy

chicken breasts in lip-smackin' barbecue sauce

lip-smackin' barbecue sauce

mahogany spice-rubbed barbecued turkey

north carolina pulled turkey barbecue

smokin' chili pepper cheeseburgers

FISH AND SHELLFISH

seared coriander halibut

crispy crunchy fish

zippy tartar sauce

fabulous foiled fish fillets

at-sa nice halibut stew

carolina crab cakes

       honey mustard sauce

shrimp de jonghe

great grilled spicy shrimp

citrus-cilantro shrimp

north carolina shrimp pilaf

thai shrimp

When I think of real meals, I think of

meat. There's nothing else so gratifying, so flavorful, so straightforward. It can handle a multitude of flavorings without being overwhelmed.

I eat meat often, which is why I always choose meats that are lean. For beef, flank steak is my cut of choice for grilling or stir-frying. Sirloin steak is even leaner, and it takes practically no time to cook. It's ideal for Lightnin' Fast Beefsteak Stew, which cooks in less than 15 minutes.

As for pork, it's much leaner than it used to be, thanks to the efforts of pork producers, who put the pigs on a diet. The leanest and most versatile pork cut of all is tenderloin, with only 15 fat grams per pound. I like to put it in a gingery marinade and then grill it. Or I make a stew with pork tenderloin, carrots and mushrooms. It makes everyone who tastes it go hog-wild. Pork tenderloin also makes good-tasting, lean breakfast sausage and Polish sausage.

Nothing is more important to keeping lean beef and pork juicy than cooking it to the proper temperature. Overcooking will make the meat dry, so the medium-rare stage is best.

Because I cooked chicken breasts so often when I was losing weight, they have to be absolutely sensational to satisfy me now. Chicken Vesuvio is redolent of olive oil and garlic, yet gets just 20 percent of its calories from fat. Chicken breasts marinated in buttermilk become extra tender and juicy; this recipe is so simple I call it E-Z. East Indian Tandoori Chicken and Thai Grilled Chicken Breasts burst with spices and are perfect for grilling.

You may never have thought of cooking a whole turkey on a grill, but it's much easier than you might think, and the results are stupendous. I rub the bird with tasty spices first and slowly grill it to a mahogany brown. And because I missed being able to indulge in the famous but fatty North Carolina "pig pickin'" barbecues, I created my own turkey barbecue using lean turkey

a guy's guide to great eating

breast cooked in a tangy, sweet and hot sauce. When you taste this, heaven waits.

Dryness can be a problem when cooking poultry, especially if you remove the fatty skin. A simple way to add moisture without fat is to immerse the bird in a saltwater brine for an hour or so before cooking. Although it may seem weird to soak a bird in a bucket of salt water, the brine makes the meat absorb water and hoard it during cooking, so the breast stays especially moist. This technique won't make the meat taste salty, and it works equally well with frozen shrimp and pork loin and tenderloin.

When I cook fish at home, I generally prepare it in the simplest way possible. Scared Coriander Halibut is a good example: I just rub it with coriander seeds and place it in an oiled skillet in the oven. While it's cooking, I make an easy nonfat sauce of vinegar, soy and lemon peel.

Whether you choose beef, pork, poultry or seafood, the recipes that follow prove you don't have to become a vegetarian to eat healthfully.

a guy's better burger

makes 6 hamburgers

My maternal grandfather, Whitmore Thomas Haynes, loved to eat. He was a big guy, even though he started his life as a two-and-a-half-pound premature baby, which earned him the nickname of Tot. My grandfather shopped at Berg's Market, in Evanston, Illinois, which had a butcher who ground his own hamburger. Hamburgers made from Berg's ground beef are the standard by which I judge all others. Few can duplicate the clean beef flavor and rich texture of those burgers.

I come very close, however, by grinding my own beef in a food processor. This way I not only can pick the cut (sirloin) and limit the fat content (to 8 percent) but also avoid potential health problems from any microbial contamination.

Through trial and error, I have learned an important lesson: I season the ground beef first and then form my burgers. Contrary to popular belief, salting the meat early in the game does not make it dry.

2 pounds boneless sirloin steak, with some fat around the edges

1 teaspoon salt

½ teaspoon fresh-ground black pepper

6 hamburger buns

1. Rinse the steak thoroughly with cold running water. Pat dry with paper towels.

2. Trim the fat from the steak and cut the fat into ½-inch chunks; set aside. Cut the remaining meat into 1-inch chunks. Weigh out a touch more than 2 ounces (⅓ cup) of the fat and discard the rest. Mix the reserved fat into the beef chunks. Refrigerate the meat mixture for a minimum of 1 hour, or until needed. (Processing warm meat and fat results in mushy burgers.)

3. **To grind:** Remove the meat mixture from the refrigerator and divide into 4 equal portions. Place one of the portions in the bowl of a food processor with the steel blade in place. Process, pulsing, for 15 (for a slightly coarse grind) to not more than 20 (for a fine grind) 1-second pulses. Transfer the meat to a large bowl and repeat with the remaining portions.

4. **To season and form:** Season the ground meat with the salt and pepper. Toss lightly with your hands to distribute the seasonings. Divide the meat into 6 equal portions and press lightly into patties with your fingertips.

5. Prepare a fire in the grill. When the coals are covered with a light ash, spread them in an even layer. Oil the grill rack, place it 5 to 6 inches over the coals and preheat the rack for 5 minutes.

6. **To cook:** Place the burgers on the rack, cover and grill to the desired doneness, 4 minutes per side for medium-rare, 5 minutes on the first side and 4 minutes on the second for medium, or 5 minutes per side for well done. Broiling under a preheated broiler or pan-grilling in a preheated pan for the same time will produce similar results.

Nutritional information per hamburger (including the bun): 353 calories (33.6% from fat), 13.2 g fat (4.8 g saturated fat), 34.6 g protein, 21 g carbohydrate, 23 mg cholesterol, 341 mg sodium.

leansuggestion: For cheeseburgers, add 4 ounces grated extra-sharp, reduced-fat cheddar cheese to the meat at the same time as the salt and pepper. (Mixing it into the meat means you can use a small amount of cheese and still get a large amount of flavor.) Proceed as directed. Each cheeseburger will have 53 more calories and 3.3 more fat grams.

rubbed and grilled flank steak

makes 4 servings

I love grilling outdoors over a real charcoal fire. My favorite grill is a Weber, since it gives me a lot of cooking control. Flank steak takes just a short time to cook and is very lean. The chili powder, garlic, cumin and Worcestershire sauce used in this rub bring out the steak's natural flavor.

1 tablespoon chili powder
1 large garlic clove, chopped and mashed
    to a paste with ½ teaspoon salt
½ teaspoon ground cumin
½ teaspoon granulated sugar
1 tablespoon plus 2 teaspoons
    Worcestershire sauce

1 flank steak (approximately 1¼
    pounds), trimmed of all visible
    fat, several shallow slits cut
    into each side

1. In a small bowl, mix together the chili powder, garlic paste, cumin and sugar, then stir in the Worcestershire sauce to make a paste.

2. Rub both sides of the steak with the paste. Put the steak into a large recloseable plastic bag, press out as much air as possible, seal the bag and chill for at least 4 hours or up to 2 days.

3. Prepare a fire in the grill. When the coals are covered with a light ash, spread them in an even layer. Oil the grill rack, place it 5 to 6 inches over the coals and preheat the rack for 5 minutes.

4.   Place the steak on the rack and grill for 5 minutes on each side for medium-rare, or 6 minutes per side for medium, or 7 minutes per side for well done. Transfer the steak to a cutting board and let stand for 5 minutes. Cut into thin slices across the grain and serve immediately.

Nutritional information per 4-ounce serving: 244 calories (42% from fat), 11.5 g fat (4.9 g saturated fat), 30.6 g protein, 2.4 g carbohydrate, 75 mg cholesterol, 422 mg sodium.

cheddar cheeseburger meat loaf

makes 8 servings

Meat loaf is the average Joe's pâté. I love it served hot with whipped potatoes and steamed green beans or cold, thinly sliced, in sandwiches.

Drained applesauce makes my meat loaf juicy. The flavor of the applesauce is almost imperceptible, and it holds in the meat's moisture. As an added benefit, the pectin from the apples helps firm up the meat loaf.

One evening, while I was assembling my meat loaf, I decided to add some reduced-fat sharp cheddar cheese, and this terrific version was born. When I serve it cold in a sandwich, I also add a slice of onion. Man, that's good eating.

¾ cup unsweetened applesauce
1 large egg
1 large egg white
⅓ cup minced onion
¼ cup chopped fresh parsley leaves
1 teaspoon salt
½ teaspoon fresh-ground black pepper
¼ teaspoon cayenne pepper
1½ pounds 93% lean ground beef

6 ounces (about 1½ cups grated) reduced-fat sharp cheddar cheese
1 cup packed fine fresh bread crumbs, from about 3 slices good-quality white sandwich bread
½ cup tomato ketchup

1. Place a strainer over a bowl deep enough so the bottom of the strainer doesn't touch the bottom of the bowl. Put the applesauce in the strainer and set aside to drain for 15 minutes; you should have ½ cup drained applesauce.

2.   Place the oven rack in the center and preheat the oven to 350 degrees. Lightly spray a 9-by-5-by-3-inch loaf pan with vegetable oil.

3.   Put the egg and egg white in a large mixing bowl and whisk until combined. Add the drained applesauce, onion, parsley, salt, black pepper and cayenne pepper and whisk until combined. Add the ground beef, cheese and bread crumbs. With clean hands, briefly combine but do not overwork.

4.   Pat the meat mixture into the prepared loaf pan, smoothing the top. Brush the ketchup over the top. Bake for 1 hour, or until a meat thermometer inserted into the center registers 160 degrees. Remove from the oven and allow to rest for 15 minutes. Serve.

Nutritional information per serving: 224 calories (36% from fat), 8.9 g fat (4.2 g saturated fat), 26.7 g protein, 9.5 g carbohydrate, 73 mg cholesterol, 725 mg sodium.

cookingtip: I use a widely available double loaf pan especially made for leaner meat loaf manufactured by Chicago Metallics (about $10). The interior pan has ridges and holes in the bottom, and an outer pan holds the fat that drains away from the meat loaf. Both pans are nonstick for quick cleanup.

saltsense: Omitting the 1 teaspoon salt reduces the sodium to 459 mg per serving.

ground beef tortilla roll-ups

makes 10 roll-ups

Before I lost weight, I enjoyed tacos overflowing with meat, cheese and sour cream. I didn't want to give up that tasty dish, so I went to work and created my slightly north-of-the-border version. I use fat-free flour tortillas and warm them in the oven instead of frying them. I use 95 percent lean ground beef to cut the fat to the bone. Instead of buying a packet full of artificial ingredients, I prepare my own seasonings. Fat-free sour cream and grated fat-free cheese provide flavor instead of fat. For a spicy boost, I chop up a couple of fresh jalapeño peppers and sprinkle some on each of my soft tacos.

2 teaspoons olive oil	1¼ cups nonfat sour cream
1½ pounds 95% lean ground beef	1 large ripe tomato, diced
1 small onion, chopped	2 cups shredded lettuce leaves
3 tablespoons tomato paste	8 ounces fat-free cheddar cheese, grated
1 tablespoon chili powder (or to taste)	
½ teaspoon Tabasco sauce	2 fresh jalapeño peppers, finely chopped (optional)
Salt to taste	
10 10-inch fat-free or low-fat flour tortillas	

1. Place the oven rack in the upper-middle position and preheat the oven to 250 degrees.

2. Place a large nonstick skillet over medium-high heat and add the oil. When it is hot, add the ground beef and onion and cook, stirring and breaking up the meat with a spoon until it loses its pink color. Drain the fat from the skillet and return it to the heat.

3. In a small bowl, whisk together the tomato paste and 3 tablespoons water until combined. Set aside.

4. Sprinkle the chili powder, Tabasco sauce and salt over the meat mixture and cook, stirring, for 1 minute, until fragrant. Push the meat to the edges of the skillet. Add the tomato paste mixture to the center of the skillet and cook for 1 minute, or until it darkens slightly. Stir into the meat. Reduce the heat to low, cover and cook for 5 minutes, until slightly thickened. Spoon into a serving bowl.

5. Meanwhile, place 2 to 4 tortillas on the oven rack, not overlapping, and bake for 2 minutes, or until soft and hot. Use a spatula to transfer them from the oven to a plate. Cover the tortillas with a double layer of paper towels. Repeat with the remaining tortillas.

6. Allow diners to assemble their own roll-ups. To assemble: lay a warm tortilla on a plate. Smear 1 tablespoon of the sour cream off-center on the tortilla. Spoon ⅓ to ½ cup of the meat mixture over the sour cream. Distribute 1 tablespoon of the diced tomato over the meat. Sprinkle some lettuce over the tomato. Sprinkle about ¼ cup cheese over the lettuce. Sprinkle some of the jalapeño peppers, if using, on top of the cheese. Fold the bottom of the tortilla up about 1 inch. From the side, roll up the tortilla.

Nutritional information per roll-up (without jalapeño peppers): 329 calories (12.5 % from fat), 4.6 g fat (1.5 g saturated fat), 27.5 g protein, 11.5 g carbohydrate, 41 mg cholesterol, 966 mg sodium.

slow-cooked pot roast with gravy

makes 6 servings, each 4 ounces; makes 2 cups gravy

My mom used to make a good pot roast from a seven-bone chuck roast and packaged onion soup mix. I wanted to create a pot roast that was less fatty and first tried top round. It was way too lean. No matter how slowly I cooked it or how low the temperature, it came out tough and as dry as sawdust.

So I went back to chuck and bought the leanest cut available: chuck arm roast. I trimmed all the visible fat and cooked it long and slow. It was rich in flavor and smooth and moist in texture. Although my pot roast is a couple of grams higher in fat than I usually allow myself, it's well worth it. When I plan to have it for dinner, I trim a few fat grams from breakfast or lunch.

roast
- 1 tablespoon olive oil
- 1 3-to-4-pound boneless chuck arm roast, trimmed of all visible fat
- 1 large onion, sliced
- 2 large garlic cloves, finely chopped
- 2 celery ribs, sliced crosswise
- 1 large or 2 medium carrots, peeled and sliced crosswise
- 1 bay leaf
- 1 teaspoon dried thyme leaves, crumbled
- ¼ teaspoon fresh-ground black pepper

gravy
- 2 tablespoons cornstarch
- ¼ teaspoon salt
  Fresh-ground black pepper to taste

1. **To make the roast:** Place the oven rack in the lower third position and preheat the oven to 300 degrees.

2. Place a Dutch oven or a large heavy-bottomed skillet over medium-high heat and add the oil. When it is hot, add the roast and lightly brown it on all sides. Transfer the roast from the Dutch oven to a plate, using large spoons so as not to pierce the meat. Set aside.

3. Add the onion and garlic to the Dutch oven and sauté for 5 to 6 minutes, or until soft. Add the celery and carrots and sauté for 3 to 4 minutes more, or until the celery turns brighter green. Add the bay leaf, thyme and pepper. Add 3 cups water, scrape up any browned bits from the bottom and bring to a boil. Remove from the heat.

4. Using the large spoons, return the roast to the Dutch oven along with any juices on the plate. Cover and place in the oven. Roast for 2½ hours, or until the meat can easily be pierced with a fork and the juices run clear. Carefully remove the cover (steam will billow out) and transfer the roast to a cutting board; let it rest for 15 minutes.

5. **Meanwhile, make the gravy:** Strain the liquid from the Dutch oven into a fat separator; discard the solids. Pour the defatted liquid into a 2-cup measuring cup, adding sufficient water to make 1¾ cups. Pour into a small saucepan and bring to a boil over medium-high heat. Whisk the cornstarch into ¼ cup water in a small bowl. When the liquid comes to a boil, add the cornstarch mixture, salt and pepper. Simmer, stirring constantly, until thickened. Remove from the heat, taste and adjust the seasonings.

6. Slice the pot roast and serve with the gravy.

Nutritional information per serving with 2 tablespoons gravy: 270 calories (35% from fat), 10.5 g fat (3.8 g saturated fat), 40.4 g protein, 0.9 mg carbohydrate, 122 mg cholesterol, 113 mg sodium.

cooking**tips**: If you don't own a fat separator, let the gravy cool and skim the fat off the top.
   ♦ If you have leftover pot roast, reheat it gently over low heat. Reheating over high heat can toughen it.

kickass beef-chunk chili

makes 12 servings

My cousin Kathy Mauer makes a chili that her five brothers crave. It's loaded with beef and beans. Kathy suggests serving the chili with homemade corn bread (page 206). A good, creamy cabbage slaw (pages 226–29) on the side completes a memorable meal.

2 tablespoons olive oil	1 28-ounce can whole tomatoes, drained (reserve liquid) and chopped
1 large onion, chopped	
1 green bell pepper, chopped	1 15.5-ounce can pinto beans, including liquid
12 garlic cloves, minced	
4 teaspoons paprika (preferably Hungarian)	1 15.5-ounce can kidney beans, including liquid
2–3 teaspoons crushed red pepper flakes	1 15.5-ounce can Great Northern beans, including liquid
2 teaspoons ground cumin	5 tablespoons cornmeal
1 teaspoon cayenne pepper	2 tablespoons all-purpose flour
1 teaspoon dried oregano, crumbled	Salt to taste
3 pounds top round, trimmed of all visible fat, cut into 1¼-inch-wide strips	

1. Bring 4 cups water to a boil in a medium saucepan.

2. Meanwhile, place a large heavy-bottomed pot over high heat and add the oil. When the oil is hot, add the onion, bell pepper and garlic. Sauté for 3 minutes, or until the vegetables begin to soften. Add the paprika, red pepper flakes, cumin, cayenne and oregano and stir constantly for 30 seconds, or until fragrant. Add the beef and cook, stirring frequently, for 3 to 4 minutes, or just until it loses its pink color; do not brown.

 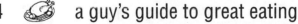

3. Add the chopped tomatoes and their liquid and the 4 cups boiling water to the beef mixture. Reduce the heat to low, cover and barely simmer, stirring occasionally, until the beef is tender, 2½ to 3 hours. (The meat should be so tender it falls apart at this point.)

4. Add all the beans and their liquid and cook for 15 minutes more, or until the beans are heated through.

5. Whisk the cornmeal and flour into 1 cup cold water and add to the chili, stirring to prevent lumps. Cook until thickened, 4 to 5 minutes. Season with salt and serve.

Nutritional information per serving (without added salt): 359 calories (18.8% from fat), 7.5 g fat (1.9 g saturated fat), 36.6 g protein, 35.4 g carbohydrate, 65 mg cholesterol, 558 mg sodium.

cookingtip: This chili freezes and reheats well.

billy's chili

makes 4 servings

Who's Billy and why is his chili recipe here? Billy is William Barton, the award-winning author of sensational science fiction books, such as *Acts of Conscience*. My wife worked with Bill, and one day he brought his homemade chili for lunch. The aroma wafting through the office was too much for Susan, and she asked for a taste. Later, Barton was generous enough to share his recipe with me.

    The cooking process is unusual, so follow the directions carefully. By doing so, you'll get a chili with a not-soon-to-be-forgotten flavor.

<table>
<tr><td>2</td><td>teaspoons olive oil</td><td>1</td><td>8-ounce can tomato sauce</td></tr>
<tr><td>1</td><td>large sweet onion, such as Vidalia or Texas Sweet</td><td>2</td><td>tablespoons apple cider vinegar</td></tr>
<tr><td>3-4</td><td>garlic cloves, minced</td><td>1</td><td>tablespoon granulated sugar</td></tr>
<tr><td>1</td><td>pound ground sirloin</td><td>1</td><td>scant tablespoon chili powder</td></tr>
<tr><td>¼</td><td>cup plus 1 teaspoon Worcestershire sauce, divided</td><td>1</td><td>teaspoon dried oregano, crumbled</td></tr>
<tr><td></td><td>Green Tabasco sauce, to taste</td><td>1</td><td>teaspoon dried basil, crumbled</td></tr>
<tr><td>1</td><td>15-ounce can cannellini (white kidney) beans, including liquid</td><td></td><td></td></tr>
</table>

1. Place a large skillet over medium-high heat and add the oil. When it is hot, add the onion and garlic and cook, stirring occasionally, for 5 to 6 minutes, or until they begin to turn golden. Put the ground sirloin on top of the onions and press it into the onions. Add ¼ cup of the Worcestershire sauce and a sprinkle of green Tabasco sauce. Cover and cook until the meat is cooked through, 5 to 6 minutes.

 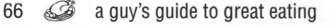

2. Meanwhile, add the beans and their liquid, tomato sauce, vinegar, sugar, chili powder, oregano, basil and the remaining 1 teaspoon Worcestershire sauce to a 5-quart saucepan. Place over medium-low heat, cover and bring to a simmer, stirring occasionally.

3. Break up the meat and, using a slotted spoon, transfer everything but the liquid to the saucepan with the bean mixture. Discard the liquid from the skillet. Simmer the chili, covered, on low heat for 1 hour. Serve.

Nutritional information per serving: 331 calories (23.7% from fat), 8.8 g fat (2.7 g saturated fat), 31.5 g protein, 29.1 g carbohydrate, 62 mg cholesterol, 658 mg sodium.

leansuggestion: Fancy Sweet Corn Bread (page 206), served steaming hot with honey, is perfect with this chili. Prepare it while the chili simmers.

saltsense: Using no-sodium tomato sauce reduces the sodium to 289 mg.

lightnin'-fast beefsteak stew

makes 6 servings

If you've ever made stew, you know that it uses tough cuts of meat and must be simmered for hours. I'm less patient than that, especially when I'm hungry. I figured stew could be speeded up by using meat that's both tender and lean. Sirloin steak has less fat than almost any other steak, and it cooks in a flash. In fact, it would get tough if simmered for hours, so this stew makes it to the dinner table in less than 30 minutes.

1 tablespoon fresh-squeezed lemon juice	¾ cup dry red wine
2¼ pounds boneless sirloin steak, trimmed of all visible fat and cut into 1-inch cubes	1½ cups beef broth, skimmed of all fat
3 tablespoons all-purpose flour	1 tablespoon paprika
4 teaspoons olive oil, *divided*	2 teaspoons salt, *divided*
1½ pounds white button mushrooms, cut into quarters	½ teaspoon fresh-ground black pepper
1 large onion, thinly sliced	1 cup frozen small peas
	1 pound dried yolkless egg noodles

1. Bring 6 quarts water to a rolling boil in a large pot.

2. Meanwhile, place the lemon juice in a medium mixing bowl. Add the sirloin cubes and toss until they are moist. Add the flour and toss until the cubes are coated.

3. Place a 6-quart saucepan over medium-high heat and add 2 teaspoons of the oil. When it is hot, add the meat and brown on all sides, about 7 minutes. Transfer the steak to a bowl and set aside.

a guy's guide to great eating

4. Add the remaining 2 teaspoons olive oil to the saucepan. Add the mushrooms and onion and sauté until soft, 6 to 7 minutes. Add the wine and simmer for 1 minute. Stir in the broth, paprika, ½ teaspoon of the salt and pepper and simmer, stirring occasionally, for 3 minutes. Return the steak and any accumulated juices to the saucepan, add the peas and cook until the meat is heated through, about 5 minutes.

5. Meanwhile, add the remaining 1½ teaspoons salt to the pot of boiling water. Add the noodles and stir until the water returns to a boil. Reduce the heat slightly and boil for 10 to 12 minutes, or until a noodle offers a little resistance when bitten. Drain the noodles well, and serve the stew over them.

Nutritional information per serving: 601 calories (16.8% from fat), 11.2 g fat (3.4 g saturated fat), 42 g protein, 72 g carbohydrate, 92 mg cholesterol, 609 mg sodium.

cooking**tip**: If you plan to have this stew for two meals, prepare only half (8 ounces) of the noodles. Cover and refrigerate the remaining stew. Prepare the rest of the noodles while reheating the leftover stew.

leansuggestion: Leftover stew is excellent reheated and served over Seemingly Sinful Fat-Free Roasted Garlic Whipped Potatoes (page 190) instead of noodles.

spicy beef and broccoli stir-fry

makes 4 servings

With a well-seasoned cast-iron skillet and all the ingredients ready next to the stove, I can create an Asian-style meal as good as I can get in a restaurant. Once the peeling and slicing are done, this dish cooks very quickly.

1 pound sirloin steak, trimmed of visible fat, cut against the grain into ¼-inch-by-¼-inch strips
2 tablespoons sesame seeds
2 large broccoli stalks
1 cup reduced-sodium beef broth
¼ cup reduced-sodium soy sauce
2 tablespoons minced, peeled fresh ginger
2 large garlic cloves, minced

4 teaspoons cornstarch
½ teaspoon crushed red pepper flakes
3 teaspoons canola oil, *divided*
1 yellow bell pepper, thinly sliced

4 cups hot cooked white rice (from 1⅓ cups raw rice)

1. Place the beef in a medium bowl, sprinkle with the sesame seeds and toss to coat. Set aside.

2. Cut the broccoli crowns into florets. Peel the stalks and slice them crosswise into thin rounds. Set aside.

3. In a small bowl, stir together the broth, soy sauce, ginger, garlic, cornstarch and crushed red pepper until the cornstarch dissolves. Set aside.

4. Place a large well-seasoned cast-iron skillet over medium-high heat and add 1½ teaspoons of the oil. When the oil is hot, add the beef and stir-fry until it loses its pink color, about 2 minutes. Using a slotted spoon, transfer it to a clean bowl and set aside.

5. Add the remaining 1½ teaspoons oil to the skillet. When it is hot, add the broccoli and bell pepper, cover and cook until the vegetables are just tender, stirring occasionally, about 3 minutes. Stir the broth mixture and add it to the skillet. Return the beef and any accumulated juices to the skillet. Cook until the sauce thickens, stirring occasionally, about 1 minute. Serve immediately over the rice.

Nutritional information per serving: 471 calories (23.2% from fat), 12.1 g fat (2.9 g saturated fat), 34.2 g protein, 56.3 g carbohydrate, 70 mg cholesterol, 891 mg sodium.

lean beef goulash

makes 6 servings, each a little more than 1 cup

The sweet onions in this goulash make the other flavors blossom. Real imported Hungarian paprika imparts the authentic taste, with vinegar and lemon juice adding spark.

1 tablespoon olive oil
1 pound sweet onions (such as Vidalia or Texas Sweets), diced (about 3 large)
2 tablespoons white wine vinegar
2 tablespoons paprika (preferably Hungarian)
2 garlic cloves, minced
½ teaspoon dried marjoram, crumbled
½ teaspoon lemon peel
½ teaspoon salt, plus more if needed
2 cups reduced-sodium beef broth, preferably homemade

4 tablespoons tomato paste
2½ pounds top round (sometimes labeled London broil), trimmed of all visible fat and cut into 1-inch cubes
½ teaspoon fresh-ground black pepper

¾ cup nonfat sour cream, *divided*
Chopped fresh dill

1. Place a 5-quart saucepan over medium-high heat and add the oil. When it is hot, add the onions and cook, stirring occasionally, until golden around the edges, about 7 minutes.

2. Add the vinegar, paprika, garlic, marjoram, lemon peel and ½ teaspoon salt. Cook, stirring constantly, until nearly dry, 1 to 2 minutes. Stir in the broth and tomato paste and bring to a simmer. Add the beef, reduce the heat to low, cover and gently simmer

a guy's guide to great eating

until it is fork-tender, about 1½ hours. Taste and add additional salt, if necessary, and the pepper. Garnish each serving with 2 tablespoons of the sour cream and sprinkle with a little fresh dill. Serve.

Nutritional information per serving: 351 calories (22.8% from fat), 8.9 g fat (2.4 g saturated fat), 47 g protein, 16.8 g carbohydrate, 113 mg cholesterol, 637 mg sodium.

leansuggestion: Serve over cooked wide yolkless egg noodles.

cookingtip: Reheat leftovers over very low heat to keep the meat tender.

 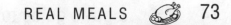

quick hamburger stroganoff

makes 6 servings

I had planned to sail right home from the office to make a tasty and healthful meal. But traffic on the interstate road was backed up for several long, hot miles, and I burst into the kitchen an hour late, tired and irritable. My wife, who arrived after I did, gave me that "What's for dinner?" look. Oh, brother.

That night, I created a version of those hamburger mixes that proliferate on the supermarket shelves. With fewer than 5 grams of fat per serving, it registers a lot lower on the fat-o-meter than the most popular commercial version, which has a hefty 13 grams. That's a big fat savings for using my noodle.

3 cups beef broth, skimmed of all fat
1 teaspoon olive oil
½ cup chopped onion
1 garlic clove, minced
1 pound 95% lean ground beef
1½ cups skim milk
1 8-ounce package dried medium egg noodles

1 tablespoon chopped fresh parsley
½ cup nonfat sour cream
1½ tablespoons cornstarch
1 tablespoon coarse Dijon mustard
¼ teaspoon fresh-ground black pepper

1. Bring the broth to a boil in a 2-quart saucepan.

2. Meanwhile, place a 10-inch nonstick skillet over medium-high heat and add the oil. When it is hot, add the onion and garlic and sauté for 2 minutes, or until just softened. Add the ground beef and cook, breaking up with the edge of a spoon, until the meat loses its pink color, 4 to 5 minutes. Drain the fat from the skillet. Add the hot broth and milk to the skillet and bring to a boil, stirring occasionally. Stir in the noo-

dles and parsley. Reduce the heat to low, cover and simmer for 5 minutes, or until a noodle offers a little resistance when bitten, stirring occasionally.

3. In a small bowl, whisk together the sour cream, cornstarch, mustard and pepper. Stir the mixture into the skillet and remove from the heat. Let stand, uncovered, for 5 minutes. Stir before serving.

Nutritional information per serving: 301 calories (13.5% from fat), 4.5 g fat (0.76 g. saturated fat), 25.6 g protein, 37.8 g carbohydrate, 60.3 mg cholesterol, 600 mg sodium.

saltsense: Two-thirds of the sodium comes from the canned beef broth. If you are on a sodium-restricted food plan, substitute reduced-sodium beef broth.

 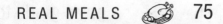

all-beef italian sausage

makes 18 ounces uncooked sausage

Some Italian sausage gets fully 80 percent of its calories from fat! The only way I can control the quality and type of ingredients is to make the sausage myself. This way, I know it's good meat and not "everything but the squeal."

My version contains lots of fennel seeds, which are what make it taste so good. The wine that further boosts the flavor is a drinkable red. Choosing lean ground beef means I decide how much fat gets in.

I use my Italian sausage for Homemade Great-Eating Pizza (page 145) and spaghetti sauce or instead of ground beef in lasagna. I also put it in stuffed peppers (page 78). Once you try this sausage, you'll never go back to store-bought.

1 pound 95% lean ground beef
¼ cup minced onion
2 tablespoons dry red wine or beef broth
2 medium garlic cloves, minced
1¼ teaspoons whole fennel seeds
1 teaspoon paprika
¾ teaspoon salt

¼ teaspoon crushed red pepper flakes, or to taste (optional)
¼ teaspoon fresh-ground black pepper
⅛ teaspoon ground bay leaf (available in grocery stores)
Pinch of dried thyme

1. Mix all the ingredients by hand in a large mixing bowl; do not overmix.

2. Lightly spray a large nonstick skillet with vegetable oil. Sauté the sausage over medium-high heat, breaking it up with a spoon, until lightly browned; drain the fat and liquid from the pan. The cooked sausage may be used as pizza topping or added to spaghetti sauce or other dishes.

Nutritional information per ounce (cooked): 45 calories (28.5% from fat), 1.4 g fat (0.5 g saturated fat), 8 g protein, 0.7 g carbohydrate, 15 mg cholesterol, 158 mg sodium.

cooking**tips**: For hot Italian sausage, add ½ teaspoon cayenne pepper with the other herbs and spices.

- The sausage may be divided into 2 equal portions. Place each portion in a recloseable plastic freezer bag, press out as much air as possible and freeze until needed; it will keep for 6 months. To defrost, remove from the freezer and thaw in the refrigerator for 12 hours, or until soft. Cook as directed.

 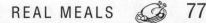

red peppers stuffed with sausage and rice

makes 4 servings

Over the last 25 years, I started trying to duplicate a favorite recipe for stuffed peppers. I didn't succeed until I discovered that using my own homemade sausage made all the difference. Are these as good as the peppers I remember? Nope. They're better.

4 medium bell peppers, preferably red
3 tablespoons minced onion
1 large garlic clove, minced
½ pound All-Beef Italian Sausage (page 76)
1 16-ounce can plum tomatoes, drained (reserve liquid) and chopped, *divided*
1½ cups hot cooked rice (from ½ cup raw rice)

½ cup frozen corn kernels, defrosted
1 ounce Parmesan cheese, freshly grated (⅓ cup)
½ teaspoon salt
¼ teaspoon fresh-ground black pepper
¼ teaspoon paprika
¼ teaspoon dried basil, crumbled

1. Place the oven rack in the lower-middle position and preheat the oven to 350 degrees. Bring a large pot of salted water to a boil.

2. Trim the stem end from the bell peppers, leaving them whole, and remove the seeds. Place the peppers in the boiling water and cook for 5 minutes. Drain well.

3. Lightly spray a large nonstick skillet with vegetable oil and place over medium-high heat. Add the onion and garlic and sauté for 1 minute, or until they just begin to soften; do not let the garlic brown. Add the sausage meat and sauté until it loses its pink

color, 3 to 4 minutes. Stir in ½ cup of the tomatoes, rice, corn, Parmesan, salt, pepper, paprika and basil and cook for 2 minutes, or until just heated through. Remove from the heat.

4.   Stuff the whole peppers with the sausage mixture. Spray an 8-by-8-by-2-inch baking dish with vegetable oil and place the peppers upright in it. Pour the remaining tomatoes and their juice around the peppers and bake for 15 minutes, or until the peppers are tender and the filling is hot. Spoon the tomato sauce from the bottom of the dish over the peppers and serve.

Nutritional information per pepper: 250 calories (20.3% from fat), 5.7 g fat (2.7 g saturated fat), 18.8 g protein, 32 g carbohydrate, 37 mg cholesterol, 797.5 mg sodium.

saltsense: Substituting no-salt-added canned tomatoes reduces the sodium to 383 mg per serving.

baked potatoes with meat sauce

makes 4 servings

One evening, I baked a couple of potatoes and created a tasty meat sauce while they were in the oven. When the potatoes were done, so was the sauce. I cut an X in the top of each potato and ladled on the sauce. It tasted great, and cleanup was a breeze. Thanks to their skins, potatoes have a healthy amount of fiber, cleverly disguised.

4 baking (russet) potatoes, scrubbed and pierced in several places with a knife

1 teaspoon olive oil

1 pound 95% lean ground beef or 93%-97% lean ground turkey breast

1 large onion, chopped

1 medium green bell pepper, chopped

1 garlic clove, minced

½ pound white button mushrooms, cleaned, stem ends trimmed and sliced

1 6-ounce can tomato paste

2 15-ounce cans tomato sauce

2 teaspoons fennel seeds, crushed

1½ teaspoons dried basil, crumbled

1 teaspoon dried oregano, crumbled

1 teaspoon clover or other mild honey

¼ teaspoon fresh-ground black pepper

¼ teaspoon crushed red pepper flakes (optional)

¼ cup fresh-grated Parmesan cheese, *divided*

1. Place the oven rack in the center and preheat the oven to 425 degrees. Place the potatoes in the oven and bake for 50 to 60 minutes, or until they give easily when pressed. Set aside.

2. Meanwhile, place a 3-quart saucepan over medium-high heat and add the oil. Add the ground beef or turkey, onion, bell pepper and garlic. Cook, stirring frequently,

until the meat loses its pink color and the onions begin to soften, about 5 minutes. Add the mushrooms and cook until they give off their liquid. Drain the fat and liquid from the pan.

3. Reduce the heat to medium and add the tomato paste and sauce. Bring to a simmer, stirring frequently, then add the fennel seeds, basil, oregano, honey, pepper and red pepper flakes. Bring to a boil, reduce the heat to low, cover and simmer for 30 minutes.

4. Place each potato in a serving bowl. Cut an X in the top of each potato and press so they open. Ladle equal amounts of sauce over each potato. Sprinkle each with 1 table-spoon Parmesan cheese. Serve.

Nutritional information per serving: 561 calories (15.8% from fat), 9.8 g fat (3.6 g saturated fat), 37 g protein, 87 g carbohydrate, 66 mg cholesterol, 1,037 mg sodium.

leansuggestion: Vegetarians will love this recipe if you make it with one of the all-vegetable ground beef substitutes, such as Morningstar Farms Burger-Style Recipe Crumbles, found in the freezer section of most supermarkets.

saltsense: Since most of the sodium in this dish comes from the tomato sauce, it can be reduced by using no-salt-added tomato sauce.

 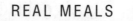

homemade jimdandy kielbasa sausage

makes 6 sausages, each 5 ounces before cooking

Kielbasa is a smoky Polish sausage. Since I originally came from the Chicago area, which has the largest Polish population outside Kraków, it made perfect sense to create a lean Old World sausage. Getting the spice mixture just right was difficult. I tested and tasted many batches before I was satisfied. My favorite way to serve this kielbasa is with steamed sauerkraut and boiled potatoes.

2 pounds pork tenderloin, trimmed of all visible fat

3 teaspoons kosher salt (or 1½ teaspoons regular salt)

4 garlic cloves, minced

2 teaspoons granulated sugar

1 teaspoon Liquid Smoke

1 teaspoon fresh-ground black pepper

1 teaspoon ground marjoram

¼ teaspoon fresh-grated nutmeg

⅛ teaspoon ground allspice

1. Cut the pork into 1-inch pieces. Place on a tray small enough to fit in the freezer and freeze for 15 minutes, or until firm. Add half the pork cubes to a food processor with the steel blade in place. Pulse until the meat is chopped into ⅛-inch pieces, about 15 one-second pulses. Transfer the pork to a large mixing bowl. Repeat with the remaining pork.

2. Add 2 tablespoons ice water and the remaining ingredients to the pork. With clean hands or wooden spoons, toss the pork and spices together until just combined; do not overmix. Place the sausage in a plastic bag, press out the air, seal and refrigerate for at least 24 hours or up to 2 days, to allow the flavors to blend.

  a guy's guide to great eating

3. With your hands, form the sausage into link shapes or patties and grill, broil or sauté in a small amount of olive oil. Serve.

Nutritional information per cooked sausage: 186 calories (29.9% from fat), 6.2 g fat (2.2 g saturated fat), 29.6 g protein, 1.0 g carbohydrate, 91 mg cholesterol, 597 mg sodium.

cooking**tip**: Liquid Smoke can be found alongside the condiments in most supermarkets.

saltsense: Omitting the salt reduces the sodium per sausage to 64 mg.

pork chops baked in sour cream

makes 4 servings

When I weighed over 300 pounds, I sautéed pork chops in bacon fat to brown them before baking. Did my pork chops have a wonderful flavor? Count on it. Were they loaded with fat? You betcha.

Today, my pork chops are lean. By using a nonstick skillet and a small amount of olive oil, I can brown my chops to increase their flavor *and* keep them healthful. I further enhance them with fresh-squeezed lemon juice and brandy. Nonfat sour cream adds creaminess to the sauce without fat.

⅔ cup nonfat sour cream
2 tablespoons fresh-squeezed lemon juice
1 teaspoon granulated sugar
½ teaspoon dried thyme, crumbled (or 1½ teaspoons chopped fresh thyme leaves)
½ teaspoon salt
¼ teaspoon fresh-ground black pepper

4 center-cut loin pork chops (4–5 ounces each), trimmed of all visible fat
About ¾ cup all-purpose flour
2 teaspoons olive oil
1 large shallot, chopped
¼ cup brandy or cognac

1. Place the oven rack in the center and preheat the oven to 350 degrees.

2. In a small bowl, whisk together the sour cream, ½ cup water, the lemon juice, sugar, thyme, salt and pepper. Set aside.

3. Dredge the pork chops in the flour, pressing the flour onto the meat; discard the remaining flour. Place a large, nonstick ovenproof skillet over medium heat and add the oil. When it is hot, add the chops and cook on both sides until golden, 5 to 6 minutes per side. Transfer the chops to a plate and set aside. Add the shallot to the

pan and cook until soft, about 4 minutes. Add the brandy or cognac and scrape up the browned bits on the bottom of the pan. Stir in the sour cream mixture. Return the chops and any accumulated juices to the pan and spoon the sauce over the chops. Cover the skillet and bake for 1 hour, or until the pork chops can easily be pierced with a fork. Serve immediately.

Nutritional information per serving: 294 calories (31.6% from fat), 10.3 g fat (1.5 g saturated fat), 33.8 g protein, 12 g carbohydrate, 99 mg cholesterol, 381 mg sodium.

cookingtip:You can substitute 3 tablespoons chopped onion and 1 minced garlic clove for the shallot.

leansuggestion: This dish is terrific served with steamed green beans and boiled potatoes.

 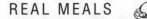

never-better roasted pork loin

makes 6 servings

For years, I shied away from pork loin because every one I had ever had was dry and tough. Because modern pigs are bred to be leaner and leaner, a juicy, moist and tender roast loin seemed impossible to achieve.

At least that was what I thought until I read an article about roasting pork loin in *Cook's Illustrated*, written by Stephen Schmidt, the author of *Master Recipes* (1998). Schmidt discovered that roasting the pork at a high temperature, then letting it rest off the heat and roasting it again at a lower temperature produced a succulent roast every time.

You'll note that the recipe starts with a chilled roast right out of the refrigerator. That's no mistake. If you try this technique with a room-temperature roast, it will be overcooked.

2 teaspoons rubbed dried sage leaves
1 teaspoon salt
1 teaspoon celery salt
1 teaspoon dry mustard (I like Colman's)
1 teaspoon fresh-ground black pepper

1 boneless center-cut pork loin roast, rolled and tied (about 2¼ pounds)

1. In a small bowl, combine the sage, salt, celery salt, mustard and pepper. Rub the spice mixture all over the roast. Wrap the roast in aluminum foil and refrigerate it for at least 2 hours or up to 3 days.

2. Place the oven rack in the center and preheat the oven to 475 degrees. Lightly spray a roasting rack with vegetable oil and place it in the center of a jelly-roll pan lined with heavy-duty foil. Remove the roast from the refrigerator, remove the foil and place the roast on the prepared rack. Roast, uncovered, for exactly 30 minutes.

3. Remove the roast from the oven. Immediately reduce the oven temperature to 325 degrees. Let the uncovered roast rest, at room temperature, for 30 minutes. Return the roast to the oven for 15 to 30 minutes, or until a meat thermometer inserted into the center registers 145 degrees.

4. Let the roast stand at room temperature, uncovered, for 20 minutes, to allow the internal temperature to rise to 150 to 155 degrees. Carve the roast into thin slices and serve immediately.

Nutritional information per 4-ounce serving: 237 calories (42.3% from fat), 10.9 g fat (3.9 g saturated fat), 32.5 g protein, 0 g carbohydrate, 92 mg cholesterol, 768 mg sodium.

cookingtip: Be sure to use a boneless roast. Using the same technique for a bone-in roast will result in undercooked, unsafe meat.

leansuggestion: Serve with Dijon mustard on the side.

saltsense: Omitting the 2 teaspoons salt reduces the sodium to 66 mg per serving.

southwestern peppery pork with white beans

makes 6 servings

In this dish, cumin, sweet onion, bell peppers and garlic play up the pork to its best advantage. It makes a terrific meal for guests and delivers only 5 fat grams per serving. That's a great way to have your guests say a heartfelt "Thank you."

1 tablespoon olive oil

1 pork tenderloin (about ¾ pound), trimmed of all visible fat and cut across the grain into ¼-by-1-inch strips

1½ teaspoons ground cumin

1 medium-large sweet onion (such as Vidalia or Texas Sweet), halved lengthwise and cut into slivers

1 large green bell pepper, cored and cut into julienne strips

1 large red bell pepper, cored and cut into julienne strips

2 garlic cloves, minced

1 medium zucchini, cut into julienne strips

1 15-ounce can cannellini beans or Great Northern beans, drained and rinsed

1 14.5-ounce can diced tomatoes, including liquid

1 4-ounce can chopped mild green chilies, drained

1 cup chopped fresh parsley leaves

2 tablespoons reduced-sodium soy sauce

½ teaspoon granulated sugar

¼ teaspoon fresh-ground black pepper

¼ teaspoon cayenne pepper, or to taste

4 cups hot cooked white rice, preferably basmati (from 1½ cups raw rice)

1. Place a large nonstick skillet over medium-high heat and add the oil. When it is hot, add the pork and sauté for 2 minutes, or just until it starts to turn gray. Sprinkle the cumin over the pork and sauté until the pork loses its pink color.

2. Add the onion, bell peppers and garlic and sauté for 3 minutes, or until the onion starts to soften. Add the zucchini and sauté for 1 minute. Add the beans, tomatoes and their juice and chilies, reduce the heat to low and simmer for 5 minutes.

3. Stir in the parsley, soy sauce, sugar, and black and cayenne peppers. Serve immediately over the rice.

Nutritional information per serving (with rice): 366 calories (12.5% from fat), 5.1 g fat (1.2 g saturated fat), 23.8 g protein, 56 g carbohydrate, 37 mg cholesterol, 510 mg sodium.

saltsense: Reducing the soy sauce to 1 tablespoon will lower the sodium to 393 mg per serving.

 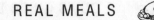

pork tenderloin with mushrooms and carrots

makes 6 servings

Cooking this tenderloin in a flavorful broth with carrots, onions and mushrooms keeps it moist. The sauce is done at the same time as the meat. It's hard to believe this dish can be so flavorful with less than 10 fat grams per serving.

3 teaspoons olive oil, *divided*
1¾ pounds pork tenderloin, trimmed of all visible fat, cut into 2-inch cubes and patted dry with paper towels
½ large onion, chopped
1 celery rib, strings removed and chopped
1 bay leaf
2 cups fat-free reduced-sodium chicken broth (preferably homemade)
4 large carrots, peeled, trimmed and cut diagonally into 1-inch pieces
½ pound white button mushrooms, cleaned, stems trimmed and thinly sliced

¼ cup all-purpose flour
½ cup nonfat sour cream
1½ teaspoons fresh-squeezed lemon juice
¼ cup minced fresh parsley leaves
1 teaspoon salt
¼ teaspoon fresh-ground black pepper

4 cups hot cooked white or brown rice (from 1⅓ cups raw rice)

1. Place a 5-quart heavy-bottomed saucepan over medium-high heat and add 2 teaspoons of the oil. When it is hot, brown the pork in batches, transferring it to a bowl as soon as it is browned. Set aside. Add the onion, celery and bay leaf and sauté for 2 minutes, until the onion just starts to soften.

2. Add the broth and 2 cups water to the saucepan, reduce the heat to low, cover and heat until steam rises from the liquid, about 5 minutes. (Do not let it boil.) Return the browned pork and any accumulated juices to the pan, add the carrots, cover and cook for 1 hour and 15 minutes, or until tender.

3. After 1 hour, place a nonstick skillet over medium heat and add the remaining 1 teaspoon oil. When it is hot, add the mushrooms and cook, stirring occasionally, until the liquid they give off has mostly evaporated. Reduce the heat to medium-low, sprinkle the mushrooms with the flour and cook, scraping up the brown bits from the bottom of the skillet, for 3 minutes. Remove from the heat and stir in the sour cream and ¼ cup of the liquid from the pork.

4. Add the mushroom mixture to the pork and cook, stirring, until the sauce thickens, about 2 minutes. Stir in the lemon juice, parsley, salt and pepper. Serve immediately over the rice.

Nutritional information per serving (with rice): 377 calories (17.4% from fat), 9.8 g fat (3.7 g saturated fat), 32.7 g protein, 44.4 g carbohydrate, 96 mg cholesterol, 584 mg sodium.

leansuggestions: You can also add 1 cup of baby peas 5 minutes before serving.
- French bread makes a great accompaniment to sop up the juices.

garlic-and-ginger-flavored grilled pork tenderloin

makes 8 servings

Pork tenderloin cooks in a flash, and it delivers tender, flavorful meat every time. This pork tenderloin is marinated in garlic, ginger and soy sauce. Lime juice and mustard add just the right amount of zing.

½ cup fat-free reduced-sodium chicken broth, *divided*
2 tablespoons cornstarch

⅓ cup fresh-squeezed lime juice
2 tablespoons reduced-sodium soy sauce
2 tablespoons grated fresh ginger
6 large garlic cloves, coarsely chopped
1 tablespoon olive oil

2 teaspoons Dijon mustard
½ teaspoon salt
¼ teaspoon fresh-ground black pepper
⅛ teaspoon cayenne pepper, or to taste

4 pork tenderloins (about ¾ pound each), trimmed of all visible fat

1. In a small bowl, whisk 1 tablespoon of the chicken broth with the cornstarch. Set aside. Bring the remaining broth to a boil in a small saucepan over high heat. Whisk in the cornstarch mixture and return to a boil. Remove from the heat and let cool.

2. Put the cooled broth mixture and the remaining ingredients, except for the pork, in a blender and blend until combined, about 15 seconds.

3. Place the tenderloins in a large plastic bag and add the marinade. Press out the excess air and seal the bag. Let the pork marinate in the refrigerator, turning occasionally, for at least 4 hours or up to 1 day. Remove from the refrigerator 30 minutes before grilling.

4. Prepare a fire in the grill. When the coals are covered with a light ash, spread them in an even layer. Oil the grill rack, place it 5 to 6 inches over the coals and preheat the rack for 5 minutes.

5. Remove the tenderloins from the marinade, letting the excess drip off. Discard the remaining marinade. Place the tenderloins on the grill rack, cover and grill for 15 to 20 minutes, turning every 5 minutes, until a meat thermometer inserted into the center registers 160 degrees.

6. Transfer the meat to a cutting board and let stand for 5 minutes. Cut across the grain into ¼-inch-thick slices and serve.

Nutritional information per serving: 204 calories (15.6% from fat), 5.8 g fat (2 g saturated fat), 35.6 g protein, 0 g carbohydrate, 111 mg cholesterol, 185 mg sodium.

lean suggestions: Serve with Sweet n' Hot Onion Marmalade (page 94).
- Want a sandwich treat? Mix 2 tablespoons cold Sweet n' Hot Onion Marmalade into 4 ounces softened nonfat cream cheese. Spread on whole-grain bread, layer on thin slices of the pork and top with shredded romaine lettuce.

sweet n' hot onion marmalade

makes about 2 cups

Once you try this marmalade on pork tenderloin, you'll never eat it plain again.

2 teaspoons olive oil
1¼ pounds sweet onions (such as Vidalia or Texas Sweets), finely chopped
2 jalapeño peppers, minced (including seeds)
2 tablespoons clover or other mild honey

3 tablespoons red wine vinegar
½ teaspoon salt
¼ teaspoon fresh-ground black pepper

1. Place a large skillet over medium heat and add the oil. When it is hot, add the onions and cook until golden, 8 to 9 minutes. Add the jalapeños and cook, stirring, for 2 minutes, or until they just start to soften.

2. Add the honey and cook, stirring, for 1 minute. Stir in the vinegar and simmer, stirring, until almost all the liquid has evaporated, 7 to 8 minutes. Add ¼ cup water and simmer, stirring, until the mixture is slightly thickened and the onions are very tender, about 10 minutes. Stir in the salt and pepper. Serve warm.

Nutritional information per tablespoon: 14.6 calories (17.6% from fat), 0.3 g fat (trace of saturated fat), trace of protein, 2.9 g carbohydrate, 0 mg cholesterol, trace of sodium.

e-z buttermilk-marinated roasted chicken breasts

makes 4 servings

This dish is as easy as it gets. Several years ago, I saw a recipe on *Bon Appétit*'s Web site for a buttermilk-marinated chicken. It sounded wonderful, so I tried it with chicken breasts, knowing they were far leaner than dark meat. The buttermilk tenderizes the meat, adds moisture and provides a tasty glaze.

I buy the chicken breasts on Saturday and marinate them until Monday evening, then roast them for a sensational supper.

4 skin-on, bone-in chicken breast halves (about 1½ pounds total), rinsed under cold water and patted dry

1 quart low-fat buttermilk
Salt and fresh-ground black pepper

1. Place the chicken breasts and buttermilk in a 1-gallon plastic bag. Press out as much air as possible, seal the bag and turn to coat the chicken. Refrigerate for at least 4 hours or up to 48 hours, turning the bag occasionally.

2. Place the oven rack in the lower-middle position and preheat the oven to 400 degrees. Place a wire rack on a jelly-roll pan. Remove the chicken breasts from the bag and place them on the rack, skin side up. Season with the salt and pepper to taste.

3. Roast for 25 to 30 minutes, or until the chicken is cooked through. Let stand for 10 minutes and serve.

Nutritional information per serving (without added salt): 187 calories (10.3% from fat), 2.2 g fat (0.6 g saturated fat), 38.8 g protein, trace of carbohydrate, 98 mg cholesterol, 111 mg sodium.

leansuggestion: Use leftovers for sandwiches, such as Classic Clubhouse Sandwich (page 256).

thai grilled chicken breasts

makes 3 servings

There are few things more satisfying than cooking outdoors on a good grill, preferably with hardwood charcoal. The very best thing is to start with chicken breasts marinated in flavorful spices.

The following mixture is misleadingly simple, but everyone who has tasted this chicken agrees that it tastes dynamite. It also makes a dandy cold chicken sandwich.

1 tablespoon granulated sugar

1 tablespoon vegetable oil

1 tablespoon plus 1 teaspoon reduced-sodium soy sauce

1 tablespoon fresh-squeezed lemon juice

1 small garlic clove, chopped

1 teaspoon fresh-ground black pepper

1 teaspoon ground cumin

1 teaspoon ground coriander

½ teaspoon turmeric

3 skin-on, bone-in chicken breast halves (about 1½ pounds total), rinsed under cold water and patted dry

1. In a medium bowl, whisk together all the ingredients except for the chicken. Put the marinade and the chicken breasts in a recloseable plastic bag, press out as much air as possible and seal. Refrigerate for at least 2 hours or up to 24 hours. Discard any unused marinade. About 45 minutes before you plan to grill, remove the chicken from the refrigerator and let it come to room temperature.

2. Prepare a fire in the grill. When the coals are covered with a light ash, spread them in an even layer. Oil the grill rack, place it 5 to 6 inches over the coals and preheat the rack for 5 minutes.

3. Sear the chicken breasts, skin side down, on the grill rack for about 2 minutes. Turn

the chicken skin side up and sear for 2 minutes more. Move the chicken away from the direct heat and grill, skin side up, covered, for 12 to 14 minutes, or until cooked through. Transfer to a serving platter. Using a paper towel for a good grip, remove the skin from the chicken and serve.

Nutritional information per serving: 252 calories (10.4% from fat), 2.4 g fat (0.8 g saturated fat), 52 g protein, 0 g carbohydrate, 132 mg cholesterol, 149 mg sodium.

leansuggestion: These chicken breasts are fabulous served with a creamy cabbage slaw (pages 226–28), corn on the cob and sliced ripe tomatoes.

east indian tandoori chicken breasts

makes 6 servings.

Back in the 1980s, when I worked in the custom photo lab business in Chicago, my friend David, a service technician, would occasionally drop in at lunchtime. We would head for a nearby Indian restaurant with a great buffet lunch. The chicken there was exotically spiced and cooked in a tandoor, a clay oven heated by charcoal to more than 500 degrees. Seared instantly on the outside, the meat remained moist inside and had a terrific flavor. This marinade has all the flavors of India, and the grill approximates the heat of a tandoor.

1 tablespoon ground cumin
2 teaspoons ground coriander
1 teaspoon cayenne pepper
1 teaspoon ground cinnamon
½ teaspoon ground cardamom
½ cup nonfat plain yogurt
    Juice of 1 lemon

1 inch fresh ginger, finely diced
1 tablespoon paprika

6 skinless, bone-in chicken breast
    halves (about 3 pounds total),
    rinsed under cold water and
    patted dry

1. Place the cumin, coriander, cayenne, cinnamon and cardamom in a small, dry sauté pan. Toast over medium heat, stirring often, until the spices start to smoke, 2 to 3 minutes. (The spices will look wet as their oils are released and will be very fragrant.) Transfer to a small bowl. Add the yogurt, lemon juice, ginger and paprika and whisk until combined.

2. Coat each chicken breast with the spice paste. Place the chicken in a recloseable plastic bag, press out as much air as possible, seal and refrigerate for at least 1 hour or up to 24 hours. About 45 minutes before grilling, remove the chicken from the refrigerator.

3. Prepare a fire in the grill. When the coals are covered with a light ash, move them to one side of the grate, using long-handled tongs. Oil the grill rack, place it 5 to 6 inches over the coals and preheat the rack for 5 minutes.

4. Place the chicken on the grill rack, near but not directly over the hot coals, and grill, turning once, taking care not to let the spice paste burn, for 16 to 20 minutes, or until cooked through. Transfer the chicken to a serving platter. Using a paper towel for a good grip, remove the skin from the chicken. Serve immediately.

Nutritional information per serving: 162 calories (19.2% from fat), 3.4 g fat (0.9 g saturated fat), 28 g protein, 3.5 g carbohydrate, 73 mg cholesterol, 80 mg sodium.

cookingtip: To cook in the oven, place the oven rack in the center and preheat the oven to 500 degrees. Spray a jelly-roll pan with vegetable oil. Place the breasts on the pan, not touching, and roast for 16 to 20 minutes, or until cooked through.

 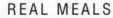

extra-crunchy country-style oven-fried chicken

makes 6 servings

Those fast-food joints sure know how to make fried chicken. The only problem is that the breading sucks up oil from the fryer, making greasy (albeit tasty) chicken.

I like to coat chicken breasts with a flavorful crunchy coating and "fry" it in the oven at a high temperature. They come out cracklin' crisp, very low in fat and so good you'll be licking your fingers.

½ cup all-purpose flour
2 teaspoons dried thyme, crumbled
1 teaspoon dried basil, crumbled
1 teaspoon dried oregano, crumbled
1 teaspoon ground cumin
1 teaspoon garlic powder
1 teaspoon fresh-ground black pepper
½ teaspoon salt
½ teaspoon curry powder
½ teaspoon cayenne pepper, or to taste

2 large egg whites
¼ cup low-fat buttermilk
2 teaspoons Dijon mustard
4 cups corn flakes
6 skinless, boneless chicken breast halves (about 3 pounds total), rinsed under cold water and patted dry

1. Place the oven rack in the lower-middle position and preheat the oven to 450 degrees. Spray a jelly-roll pan with vegetable oil.

2. Place the flour, thyme, basil, oregano, cumin, garlic powder, pepper, salt, curry powder and cayenne in a 1-quart recloseable plastic bag. Seal and shake until combined. Set aside.

3. In a small bowl, whisk together the egg whites, buttermilk and mustard. Set aside.

4. Place the corn flakes in a food processor with the steel blade in place and process, pulsing, until broken up but not turned into crumbs. Place in a medium bowl.

5. One at a time, place each chicken breast in the seasoning bag and shake until coated. Then dip it into the buttermilk mixture and then into the corn flakes, firmly pressing the corn flakes onto the chicken breast. Place each chicken breast, not touching, on the jelly-roll pan. Spray the chicken lightly with vegetable oil.

6. Bake for 20 minutes, or until the coating is golden and the chicken is cooked through. Serve immediately.

Nutritional information per serving: 289 calories (8.2% from fat), 2.7 g fat (0.6 g saturated fat), 40.8 g protein, 21.8 g carbohydrate, 98 mg cholesterol, 534 mg sodium.

saltsense: Omitting the salt reduces the sodium to 357 mg per serving.

cookingtip: This chicken stays crunchy for only a short time after it has been removed from the oven.

leansuggestions: Serve with Real American Creamy Potato Salad (page 230) and sliced ripe tomatoes.

- This chicken is great served cold at a picnic. Once the breasts are cooked, let cool to room temperature on a wire rack. Place the chicken in a plastic bag and refrigerate until needed. When you leave home, carry them in an ice-filled cooler. They will not be crunchy but will still taste good.
- Fat-free saltine cracker crumbs may be substituted for the corn flakes.

chicken with olives and peppers

makes 4 servings

I once feared that I would have to give up olives forever to maintain my weight loss of more than 100 pounds, because Dr. Dean Ornish puts avocados and olives off limits in his books about reversing heart disease.

I've since learned that using just a few olives in a dish delivers great flavor and not much fat. This dish has less than 10 fat grams per serving, with less than 17 percent of the calories coming from fat.

1 tablespoon olive oil
1 large onion, coarsely chopped
1 large garlic clove, minced
4 skinless, boneless chicken breast halves, cut into ¾-inch cubes
1 large green bell pepper, cut into 1-inch squares
½ pound white button mushrooms, cleaned, stems trimmed and thinly sliced
1 teaspoon dried basil, crumbled

½ teaspoon fresh-ground black pepper
4 medium baking (russet) potatoes, cut into 1-inch cubes
1 28-ounce can crushed plum tomatoes, including liquid
2 tablespoons fine-chopped fresh parsley leaves
12 black olives (preferably kalamata), pitted and quartered

1. Place a 5-quart pot over medium-high heat and add the oil. When it is hot, add the onion and garlic and cook, stirring, for 2 minutes. Add the chicken and bell pepper and cook, stirring, for 3 minutes. Add the mushrooms, basil and pepper and cook, stirring, for 2 minutes more. Add the potatoes and cook, stirring, for 2 minutes.

 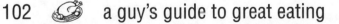

2. Add the tomatoes and their juice and the parsley, reduce the heat to medium, cover and cook, stirring occasionally, for 15 minutes. Add the olives, and cook until the potatoes are tender, about 15 minutes more. Serve.

Nutritional information per serving: 538 calories (16.6% from fat), 9.9 g fat (1.8 g saturated fat), 36 g protein, 79 g carbohydrates, 73 mg cholesterol, 1,008 mg sodium.

saltsense: Substituting no-salt-added caned tomatoes reduces the sodium to 256 mg per serving.

leansuggestion: For a tasty twist, substitute an equal amount of sweet potatoes for the russets. They add a wonderful color and a terrific sweet flavor.

 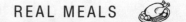

chicken vesuvio

makes 4 servings

Whenever Chicken Vesuvio floated by me in Chicago's Italian restaurants, my mouth would water from the tantalizing aroma of garlic and oregano. I wished I could order it, but the chicken and potatoes were awash in an ocean of butter and olive oil.

Chicken Vesuvio is a Chicago invention, and restaurateurs are typically tight-lipped about their special recipes. Nonetheless, I persevered and finally obtained one from someone who made me promise not to tell anyone where I got it. After considerable effort, I figured out how to remove more than 75 grams of fat.

½ cup fresh parsley leaves
2 teaspoons dried oregano, crumbled
4 large garlic cloves
2 tablespoons olive oil
4 large baking (russet) potatoes, peeled, halved crosswise, each half quartered lengthwise into thick fingers

4 skinless, bone-in chicken breast halves, rinsed under cold water and patted dry
1 teaspoon salt
½ teaspoon fresh-ground black pepper, or to taste
⅓ cup dry white wine

1. Place the oven rack in the lower middle and preheat the oven to 425 degrees.

2. Place the parsley and oregano in the work bowl of a food processor with the steel blade in place. With the processor running, add the garlic through the feed tube and process until minced. Set aside.

3. Place a large heavy-bottomed ovenproof skillet over medium-high heat and add the oil. When it is hot, add the potatoes in a single layer. Cook until they just begin to brown, about 3 minutes per side. Add the chicken and cook for 4 minutes, shaking the skillet frequently.

4. Transfer the skillet to the oven and bake for 20 minutes. Turn the chicken and potatoes over. Season with the salt and pepper. Sprinkle with the garlic mixture and wine, tossing gently to combine. Bake for 10 minutes more, or until the potatoes can be easily pierced with a knife and the chicken is cooked through. Transfer to a warm platter and serve.

Nutritional information per serving (with no added salt): 375 calories (20.4% from fat), 8.5 g fat (1.3 g saturated fat), 29.8 g protein, 40 g carbohydrate, 68 mg cholesterol, 624 mg sodium.

 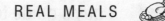

sizzlin' szechuan chicken

makes 4 servings

Szechuan is a Chinese province where spicy food is prized. My only problem with this cuisine is the amount of oil splashed into the wok during stir-frying. My recipe is low in fat, yet tastes as good as any restaurant version.

marinade and chicken

- 1 tablespoon reduced-sodium soy sauce
- 1 tablespoon cornstarch
- ½ teaspoon granulated sugar
- 1 garlic clove, minced
- 1 whole skinless, boneless chicken breast (about 10 ounces), cut into thin strips

sauce

- 1 cup fat-free reduced-sodium chicken broth
- 3 tablespoons reduced-sodium soy sauce
- 4 teaspoons cornstarch
- ½ teaspoon crushed red pepper flakes
- 1 tablespoon toasted sesame seed oil, *divided*

vegetables

- 1¾ cups coarsely chopped onions
- 2 medium carrots, peeled and cut into ⅛-inch-thick diagonal slices
- 2 small zucchini, ends trimmed, halved lengthwise, cut into ¾-inch-thick diagonal slices

- 3 cups hot cooked long-grain white rice (from 1 cup raw rice)

1. **To marinate the chicken:** In a medium bowl, whisk together the marinade ingredients until the sugar dissolves. Add the chicken and set aside to marinate for 10 to 30 minutes.

2. **To make the sauce:** In a small bowl, whisk the sauce ingredients together until the cornstarch dissolves. Set aside.

3. **To stir-fry the vegetables and chicken:** Place a large, well-seasoned cast-iron skillet over medium-high heat and add 1 teaspoon of the sesame seed oil (it will smoke). Add the chicken and stir-fry until it is opaque, 2 to 3 minutes. Transfer from the skillet to a clean bowl.

4. Add the remaining 2 teaspoons oil to the skillet. Add the onions and carrots and stir-fry for 3 minutes, or until soft. Add the zucchini and stir-fry for 1 minute more, until it turns bright green. Return the chicken to the skillet and add the sauce. Cook, scraping up the browned bits from the bottom, until the sauce thickens, about 1 minute. Serve immediately over the rice.

Nutritional information per serving (with rice): 337 calories (12.8% from fat), 4.8 g fat (0.8 g saturated fat), 22.5 g protein, 50.4 g carbohydrate, 41 mg cholesterol, 580 mg sodium.

cooking**tips**: If you don't like spicy food, reduce or omit the crushed red pepper.
- If available, use sweet onions (such as Vidalia, Maui or Texas Sweets).

succulent sunday supper roast chicken

makes 4 servings

What's the best way to bump up the moisture in chicken without adding fat? Good ole salt-water brine. I first learned about this technique in Shirley Corriher's *CookWise* (1997). The best salt for this is kosher salt or sea salt, which has a less bitter taste than iodized salt.

My brined chicken is plump, juicy, extra-golden and not at all salty, with a flavor that's out of this world.

¾ cup kosher salt
¾ cup granulated sugar
1 4-pound broiler-fryer chicken
   (not kosher)
2 medium onions, quartered
3 celery ribs, cut into 1-inch chunks

2 medium carrots, peeled and
   cut into 1-inch chunks
Fresh-ground black pepper
2 cups fat-free reduced-sodium
   chicken broth

1. Place 1 quart water and the salt and sugar in a 1-gallon recloseable plastic bag. Seal the bag and shake until the sugar and salt dissolve. Remove the bag of giblets from the cavity (reserve for another purpose or discard) and rinse the chicken, inside and out, under cold water. Place the chicken in the brine bag. Press out as much air as possible, seal the bag and refrigerate for 1½ hours or up to 24 hours.

2. Place the oven rack in the lower-middle position and preheat the oven to 375 degrees. Place a V-shaped or ordinary roasting rack in a roasting pan and lightly spray the pan and rack with vegetable oil.

3. Spread out the vegetables in the bottom of the pan underneath the V-shaped rack or around the edge of the ordinary rack. Remove the chicken from the brine bag, rinse under cold water and pat dry. Place it on the rack, back side up, and season with the pepper. Roast, basting with the broth every 10 to 12 minutes for 40 minutes. Turn it breast side up and roast and baste for 40 minutes more, or until an instant-read thermometer inserted into the breast registers 155 degrees. Let rest for 15 minutes. Remove and discard the skin and carve the chicken into serving pieces. Serve immediately.

Nutritional information per serving (equal amounts of white and dark meat): 265 calories (21.9% from fat), 6.4 g fat (1.6 g saturated fat), 48.5 g protein, 0 g carbohydrate, 155 mg cholesterol, 358 mg sodium.

cookingtips: Do not use kosher chicken. It's already spent time in a brine bath.
◆ With a slotted spoon, remove the vegetables from the bottom of the roasting pan and discard. Skim all the fat from the liquid and use to make fat-free gravy, thickened with cornstarch.

leansuggestion: Serve with Fat-Free Sour Cream Chicken Giblet Gravy (page 110).

fat-free sour cream chicken giblet gravy

makes about 3 cups

A Sunday roast chicken dinner just doesn't feel right without gravy dripping in rivulets down a pile of mashed potatoes. Giblet gravy is best, but most versions are high in fat and calories.

     The broth for my gravy is flavored with giblets. But for the gravy itself, I put in neck meat, which has little fat, and the meat from two wings in the gravy itself. Adding fat-free sour cream boosts the flavor and makes the gravy creamy.

3 cups fat-free reduced-sodium chicken broth
  Giblets from 1 chicken, rinsed under cold water
1 chicken neck, rinsed under cold water
2 chicken wings, rinsed under cold water
1 medium carrot, peeled and chopped

1 celery rib, chopped
1 tablespoon chopped onion
¼ cup all-purpose flour
½ cup fat-free sour cream
  Salt and fresh-ground black pepper, to taste

1. Place the chicken broth in a medium saucepan and bring to a boil. Add the giblets, neck, wings, carrot, celery and onion. Return to a boil, reduce the heat to low and simmer for 1 hour, or until the giblets, neck and wings are tender. Remove and discard the giblets. Transfer the neck and wings to a colander and set aside until cool enough to handle. Skim the fat from the broth.

2. Remove as much meat as possible from the chicken neck and wings, discarding the bones and skin. Chop the meat and set aside.

3. Put the flour in a medium saucepan over medium heat. Stir and shake the pan until the flour begins to turn golden brown, taking care not to burn it. Remove from the

heat. Whisk 2 cups of the broth (add water to make 2 cups, if necessary) into the browned flour and return to the heat. Add the neck and wing meat and stir until the gravy comes to a boil. Remove from the heat and whisk in the sour cream. Taste and season with the salt and pepper. Serve immediately.

Nutritional information per ¼ cup (no salt added): 32 calories (11% from fat), 0.4 g fat (0.1 g saturated fat), 2.4 g protein, 4.5 g carbohydrate, 5 mg cholesterol, 111 mg sodium.

lean suggestion: This recipe may also be used to make turkey giblet gravy. Use the turkey giblets and neck (omit the wings) and prepare the gravy as directed. I like to add 1 teaspoon Kitchen Bouquet or Gravy Master to turkey gravy just before serving.

chicken breasts in lip-smackin' barbecue sauce

makes 6 servings

This may be the best "barbecued" chicken you've ever tasted—and you can have it without the hassle of firing up the grill. The chicken ends up moist and tender, full of the terrific flavor of the sauce.

4 cups Lip-Smackin' Barbecue Sauce (opposite)	6 skinless bone-in chicken breast halves (about 3 pounds total), rinsed under cold water and patted dry

Place the barbecue sauce in a large saucepan and bring to a simmer over medium heat. Add the chicken breasts. When the sauce returns to a simmer, reduce the heat to low and simmer for 40 minutes, or until the chicken is cooked through. Remove the chicken from the sauce and serve immediately, passing the sauce at the table.

Nutritional information per serving: 220 calories (10.4% from fat), 2.6 g fat (0.6 g saturated fat), 42.6 g protein, 3.3 g carbohydrate, 106.8 mg cholesterol, 215 mg sodium.

lean suggestion: To glaze the chicken, set the oven rack 6 inches below the heat source and preheat the broiler. Line a broiler pan with foil. When the chicken is almost done, about 35 minutes, remove it from the saucepan and place the pieces, skinned side up, on the broiler pan. Broil for 2 to 4 minutes, watching carefully so the sauce doesn't burn.

lip-smackin' barbecue sauce

makes 4 cups

In the South, where I now live, strong coffee is used to enhance the flavor and color of gravy. Why not use it to do the same in a barbecue sauce? This sauce is also excellent with grilled or broiled pork tenderloin. Yee-haw, what a sauce!

2 teaspoons olive oil
2 cups chopped sweet onions (such as Vidalia or Texas Sweet)
1 tablespoon minced garlic
1 cup brewed strong coffee
1 cup Worcestershire sauce

1 cup tomato ketchup
½ cup cider vinegar
½ cup packed dark brown sugar
¼ cup chopped canned mild green chilies
2 tablespoons chili powder

1. Place a 4-quart saucepan over medium-high heat and add the oil. When it is hot, add the onions and garlic and sauté until softened, 4 to 5 minutes. Reduce the heat to medium and whisk in the remaining ingredients. Bring to a boil, reduce the heat to low and simmer, stirring occasionally, for 30 minutes. Let cool.

2. In a blender or food processor, puree the sauce in batches until smooth. Use the sauce to baste meat or poultry during the last quarter of cooking, reserving some sauce for passing at the table. Store any remaining sauce, covered, in the refrigerator for up to 2 weeks.

Nutritional information per ¼ cup: 64 calories (12.1% from fat), 0.8 g fat (0 g saturated fat), 0.3 g protein, 13.1 g carbohydrate, 0 mg cholesterol, 377 mg sodium.

mahogany spice-rubbed barbecued turkey

makes 12 servings

The best turkey I ever tasted came out of a barbecue, not an oven. The skin was a magnificent mahogany brown, and the meat had a unique flavor. I always use a fresh bird if I can get my hands on one, since it always ends up moister than a frozen one. Then I rub a special spice mixture on the outside. Barbecued turkey is super healthful: much of the fat runs out of the turkey and into a pan underneath it.

Let's see, a mahogany-colored, moister, more flavorful, leaner turkey: is there anything wrong with this picture? Yup, it'll all be gone far sooner than you'll want it to be.

1 12-pound fresh turkey (or frozen, fully defrosted)
3 tablespoons kosher salt
5 teaspoons dry mustard (I like Colman's)
1 tablespoon coarse-ground black pepper
2 teaspoons dried thyme, crumbled

2 teaspoons dried oregano, crumbled
2 teaspoons ground coriander
2 teaspoons celery salt

Canola oil

1. About 1 hour 15 minutes before you plan to grill, remove the giblets from the cavity (reserve for another purpose or discard). Rinse the turkey, inside and out, under cold water and pat dry with paper towels.

2. Stir together the salt, mustard, pepper, thyme, oregano, coriander and celery salt in a small bowl. Place the turkey on a jelly-roll pan. Brush it with the oil. Sprinkle the spice rub over the turkey and massage it into the skin. Let the bird sit for 1 hour.

3. After about 35 minutes, prepare the grill. Open all the vents. Remove the grill rack. Place 50 to 60 briquettes in a pyramid-shaped pile in the center of the lower grate. Light the briquettes, and after about 20 minutes, when a light ash forms, place half of the briquettes on one side of the grate and half on the other, using long-handled tongs. Place a 13-by-9-inch foil drip pan in the center of the grate. Put the grill rack back on the grill, making certain the handle holes are over the piles of briquettes.

4. Place the turkey, breast side up, on the rack directly above the drip pan. Cover the grill, leaving all the vents open. To maintain the proper temperature, add 6 to 8 briquettes to each side every hour. A 12-pound turkey will take about 2 hours. Check for doneness: insert an instant-read thermometer into the center of the thigh (don't let it touch the bone). It should register 180 degrees, and the breast should register 160 degrees. Place the turkey on a cutting board and let it rest for 10 minutes. Remove and discard the skin, carve and serve.

Nutritional information per 6-ounce serving (equal amounts of white and dark meat): 255 calories (15.8% from fat), 4.5 g fat (1.5 g saturated fat), 50 g protein, 0 g carbohydrate, 166 mg cholesterol, 114 mg sodium.

cookingtips: Never defrost a turkey at room temperature because of the danger of bacterial contamination. The safest way to defrost is in the refrigerator. A 12-pound turkey will take about 48 hours to defrost.

  ◆ If you choose a fresh turkey, check the "sell by" date and buy the turkey one to two days before you plan to grill it.

north carolina pulled turkey barbecue

makes 16 servings

There's a good reason that North Carolina barbecue is so famous: it tastes great! And central North Carolina barbecue sauce is different from all other barbecue sauces: it's based on vinegar instead of tomatoes or molasses, so it is tangy, sweet and hot at the same time.

Most barbecues start with a fatty pig. Instead, I created a turkey barbecue. I slowly cook a bone-in turkey breast in the barbecue sauce, then shred the meat and simmer it until it falls apart. Every North Carolinian who tastes this dish is astounded to discover that it isn't made with pork.

Since it takes a long time to make, save this dish for a large group. A word of warning, though: it will disappear fast, and you'll never have any leftovers.

2 large onions, finely chopped	2 teaspoons salt
2 cups cider vinegar	1 4½-to-5-pound skinless, bone-in
½ cup tomato ketchup	turkey breast, rinsed under
3 tablespoons Worcestershire sauce	cold water
2 tablespoons butter	1 teaspoon Liquid Smoke
2 tablespoons Tabasco sauce (or more, if	
you can stand the heat)	16 hearty sandwich rolls
2 tablespoons light brown sugar	About 1 cup low-fat cabbage
1 tablespoon fresh-ground black pepper	slaw, such as Carolina Slaw
1 ½-ounce packet Butter Buds	(page 226)
1 large garlic clove, minced	

1. In a heavy 8-quart pot, combine the onions, vinegar, ketchup, Worcestershire sauce, butter, Tabasco sauce, brown sugar, pepper, Butter Buds, garlic and salt. Bring to a simmer over medium-high heat. Reduce the heat to low and simmer for 15 minutes.

2.   Add the turkey breast to the pot, skinned side up, and simmer, covered, for 2½ hours, or until a meat thermometer inserted into the center registers 155 degrees. (Do not let the thermometer touch the bone.)

3.   Transfer the breast to a cutting board and set aside until it is cool enough to handle. Following the grain, pull off long, thin shreds of meat from the breast. Discard the bone.

4.   Stir the shredded turkey and Liquid Smoke into the sauce. Simmer over low heat, stirring occasionally, for 1½ hours, or until the meat almost falls apart. Taste and adjust the seasonings with additional salt, pepper or Tabasco sauce.

5.   Place ¾ cup of the turkey mixture on each of the sandwich rolls. Top with a tablespoon of slaw and serve.

Nutritional information per serving (with 1 tablespoon slaw): 311 calories (13.3% from fat), 4.6 g fat (1.1 g saturated fat), 32.8 g protein, 31.8 g carbohydrate, 75 mg cholesterol, 780 mg sodium.

smokin' chili pepper cheeseburgers

makes 8 servings

When I was growing up, my parents punished my brothers and me for saying bad words by sprinkling cayenne pepper on our tongues. Ouch! For many years, I wouldn't eat spicy food. I finally got over the trauma, and now I crave heat. This recipe makes a blazing burger, just the way I like it. If you prefer, leave out the jalapeño slices pressed onto each burger.

2 cups hickory chips

⅓ cup fine-chopped scallions, including the green portion

3 tablespoons nonfat plain yogurt

2 tablespoons fine-chopped jalapeño pepper, including the seeds

½ teaspoon fresh-ground black pepper

2 pounds 92% lean ground turkey breast

6 ounces reduced-fat sharp cheddar cheese, coarsely grated (about 1½ cups)

4 jalapeño peppers, sliced into ¹⁄₁₆-inch-thick rounds

8 kaiser rolls, split and toasted
Leaf lettuce
Sliced ripe tomato

1. At least 1 hour before grilling, soak the hickory chips in warm water to cover.

2. Meanwhile, whisk together the scallions, yogurt, chopped jalapeño and pepper in a medium bowl. Add the ground turkey and cheese. With clean hands, mix thoroughly, but do not overmix. Shape the mixture into eight 4-ounce patties about ¾ inch thick. Press the jalapeño slices onto each side of the burgers.

3. Prepare a fire in the grill. When the coals are covered with a light ash, arrange them around a drip pan. Drain the hickory chips and place them on top of the coals. Place the burgers on the grill rack above the drip pan, cover and grill for 10 minutes,

or until an instant-read thermometer inserted into the centers registers 160 degrees. Serve on the rolls with the lettuce and tomato.

Nutritional information per serving: 358 calories (38.6% from fat), 15.4 g fat (4.9 g saturated fat), 30.5 g protein, 22.3 g carbohydrate, 90 mg cholesterol, 507 mg sodium.

leansuggestion: Omitting the cheese reduces the calories of each burger to 298 (35% from fat) and reduces the fat to 11.6 grams (2.6 g saturated fat). Using leaner ground turkey will reduce the fat and calories even more.

 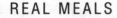

seared coriander halibut

makes 4 servings

My brother Tom is an executive chef, and I always learn at least one new technique from him at family get-togethers. When Tom heard that I was writing this cookbook, he called and gave me this recipe.

2 tablespoons coriander seeds, crushed or coarsely ground, *divided*

4 4-to-6-ounce halibut fillets, skin removed, rinsed under cold water and patted dry

Salt and fresh-ground black pepper to taste

2 teaspoons olive oil, *divided*

sauce

¼ cup balsamic vinegar

¼ cup reduced-sodium soy sauce

Peel from ½ lemon

1. Place the oven rack in the center and preheat the oven to 350 degrees.

2. Press ¾ teaspoon of the crushed coriander seeds onto each side of each halibut fillet. Season the fillets with salt and pepper.

3. Place an ovenproof nonstick skillet large enough to hold the fillets in a single layer over medium-high heat and add 1 teaspoon of the oil. When the oil is hot, add the fillets and cook until the coriander seeds are browned and the fillets are golden, 4 to 5 minutes. Add the remaining 1 teaspoon oil to the skillet, turn the fillets over and place the skillet, uncovered, in the oven. Bake for 5 minutes, or until the fish offers resistance when pressed with the back of a spoon; do not overcook.

4.   **Meanwhile, make the sauce:** Place the vinegar, soy sauce and lemon peel in a small nonreactive saucepan over medium-low heat until it begins to steam; do not boil.

5.   Pour 1 tablespoon of the sauce onto each of 4 dinner plates and place a fillet in the center of the sauce. Serve immediately.

Nutritional information per 6-ounce serving: 223 calories (26% from fat), 6.5 g fat (0.9 g saturated fat), 37 g protein, 3.1 g carbohydrate, 54 mg cholesterol, 621 mg sodium.

cooking**tip**: To crush coriander seeds, place them on a cutting board and press with the edge of a small heavy skillet to crush them. Or, place the seeds in a recloseable plastic bag, press out as much air as possible and seal. Place the bag on a cutting board and press down hard with a rolling pin. Or, empty your pepper mill. Set the grind to very coarse and add the coriander seeds. Grind the seeds until the pepper mill is empty.

leansuggestion: Serve with Special Mashed Potatoes (page 188) and Asparagus with Parmesan Cheese (page 215).

crispy crunchy fish

makes 4 servings

Frozen fish sticks taste like the box they come in, and tartar sauce is astronomically high in fat. My recipe gives fresh fish fillets a crunchy exterior while keeping them moist inside. I serve this with my own *Zippy Tartar Sauce* (opposite).

1   large egg
1   teaspoon Dijon mustard
¼   teaspoon salt
1½   cups corn flake crumbs

4   6-to-8-ounce fish fillets, fresh or thawed frozen (use cod, flounder, sole, haddock, scrod, grouper or halibut), rinsed under cold water and patted dry
     Lemon wedges

1. Place the oven rack in the lower-middle position and preheat the oven to 425 degrees. Lightly spray a jelly-roll pan with vegetable oil and set aside.

2. In a medium bowl, whisk together the egg, 1 tablespoon water, the mustard and salt. Spread the corn flake crumbs on a plate.

3. Dip each fillet into the egg mixture, letting the excess drain back into the bowl. Completely coat each fillet with the crumbs. Place on the prepared pan and lightly spray each one with olive oil. Bake for 10 minutes per inch of thickness, measured at the thickest part, turning the fillets over halfway through the cooking time, until the centers offer resistance when pressed. Serve with the lemon wedges.

Nutritional information per serving (for cod): 239 calories (10.3% from fat), 2.8 g fat (0.7 g saturated fat), 38 g protein, 12.4 g carbohydrate, 139 mg cholesterol, 440 mg sodium.

zippy tartar sauce

makes 2 cups

This is a great fiery sauce to serve with oven-fried fish.

1¾ cups low-fat mayonnaise (1 fat gram
    per tablespoon)
1 tablespoon chopped scallion, white
    part only
2 tablespoons Dijon mustard
2 tablespoons fine-chopped dill pickle (or
    dill pickle relish)
1 tablespoon small capers, drained and
    rinsed

1 teaspoon Worcestershire sauce
½ teaspoon reduced-sodium soy
    sauce
¼ cup fine-chopped fresh parsley
2 tablespoons chopped fresh dill
½ teaspoon cayenne pepper

Place all the ingredients in a food processor with the steel blade in place. Pulse several times until well combined. Place in a small bowl, cover and refrigerate for a few hours to allow the flavors to blend.

Nutritional information per tablespoon: 24 calories (39.6% from fat), 1.1 g fat (trace of saturated fat), trace of protein, 3.7 g carbohydrate, 0 mg cholesterol, 175 mg sodium.

fabulous foiled fish fillets

makes 4 servings

When I was a Boy Scout, my troop would go camping in the fall and again in the spring. Each scout was responsible for preparing his own food. A common way to make dinner was to wrap potatoes, meat and green beans in aluminum foil and toss it in the fire to cook. It tasted OK—well, even if it didn't, I ate it.

Now I use a similar technique with fish that locks in the flavor. I sauté some onion, garlic, green peppers and mushrooms in a touch of olive oil, adding some tomatoes. Then I assemble my foil packets. The result: perfectly cooked fish.

2 teaspoons olive oil
1 medium onion, thinly sliced
2 cups thin-sliced white button mushrooms
1 large green bell pepper, cut into thin strips
1 garlic clove, minced
1 cup peeled, cubed tomato (or canned plum tomatoes)

1 teaspoon fresh thyme, chopped (or ¼ teaspoon dried, crumbled)
½ teaspoon salt
⅛ teaspoon cayenne pepper
1 bay leaf
Fresh-ground black pepper
2 pounds fish fillets (sea bass, cod, flounder or halibut), cut into 4 equal pieces, rinsed under cold water and patted dry

1. Place the oven rack in the center and preheat the oven to 500 degrees. Cut heavy-duty aluminum foil into four 18-inch squares. Set aside.

2. Place a large nonstick skillet over medium-high heat and add the oil. When it is hot, add the onion, mushrooms, bell pepper and garlic. Sauté, stirring, until the

onions and peppers soften, 4 to 5 minutes. Add the tomato, thyme, salt, cayenne, bay leaf and a few grinds of pepper and cook until heated through, about 3 minutes. Set aside.

3. Spray 1 side of each piece of aluminum foil with vegetable oil. Place 1 fillet slightly off center on each piece of foil. Remove the bay leaf from the sauce and spoon one-fourth of the tomato mixture over each. Fold the foil over the fillets, roll it up and crimp the 3 open sides. Arrange the packets on a large baking sheet and bake for 10 minutes.

4. Cut open the packets (carefully, since steam will be released) and place the fish and vegetables on serving plates. Or serve the packets on the plates and open them at the table.

Nutritional information per serving (with cod): 242 calories (15.5% from fat), 4.1 g fat (0.6 g saturated fat), 42.3 g protein, 6.9 g carbohydrate, 99 mg cholesterol, 397 mg sodium.

 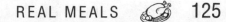

at-sa nice halibut stew

makes 6 servings

This stew is easy to make and tastes phenomenal. You don't have to make fish broth, because the recipe uses bottled clam juice. If your fishmonger will remove the skin from the fillets, all you have to do is cut them into 1-inch squares. It's hard to believe that something this tasty has less than 6 fat grams per serving. Now that is *really* nice.

1 tablespoon olive oil	½ bay leaf
1 cup chopped onion	2 baking (russet) potatoes (about 1 pound total), peeled and cut into 1-inch cubes
¾ cup chopped celery	
⅓ cup chopped green bell pepper	
2 garlic cloves, minced	2 pounds halibut fillets, skin removed, cut into 1-inch pieces
1 28-ounce can crushed tomatoes	
2 cups bottled clam juice, *divided*	1 tablespoon cornstarch
3 tablespoons fresh-squeezed lemon juice	1 tablespoon fine-chopped fresh parsley leaves
½ teaspoon fresh-ground black pepper	
¼ teaspoon dried marjoram, crumbled	

1. Place a 5-quart heavy-bottomed saucepan over medium heat and add the oil. When it is hot, add the onion, celery, bell pepper and garlic and cook, stirring, until softened, about 5 minutes. Add the tomatoes, 1¾ cups of the clam juice, lemon juice, pepper, marjoram and bay leaf. Reduce the heat to low and simmer, covered, for 30 minutes.

2. Stir in the potatoes and simmer, covered, for 30 minutes, or until they offer a touch of resistance when pierced with a knife.

3. Add the halibut. Cover and cook for 10 minutes, or until the halibut is opaque.

4. Meanwhile, in a small bowl, whisk the cornstarch with the remaining ¼ cup clam juice. When the halibut is opaque, stir the cornstarch mixture into the stew and cook until slightly thickened, about 30 seconds. Discard the bay leaf. Serve immediately, sprinkled with the parsley.

Nutritional information per serving: 321 calories (16% from fat), 5.7 g fat (0.9 g saturated fat), 35.5 g protein, 30.7 g carbohydrate, 48 mg cholesterol, 689 mg sodium.

cookingtip: You don't have baking potatoes in the house? You can go ahead and substitute red potatoes or other boiling potatoes.

leansuggestion: Warm French bread is a perfect accompaniment to sop up all the wonderful juices.

carolina crab cakes

makes 16 crab cakes

Crabmeat is a winner when it comes to fat, averaging less than 5 fat grams per pound. The problem with traditional crab cakes isn't the crab, but the binder and the oil in which it is cooked. My solution is to use a very low-fat mayonnaise and egg whites for some of the eggs. Then, instead of sautéing the crab cakes in butter, I spray them with butter-flavored vegetable oil and broil them until they are golden brown. I have tested this recipe many times, tweaking it until the balance of flavors is just right.

The story is that crab cakes originated in Maryland, but since I'm a Carolina guy, these are Carolina crab cakes. Sorry, Maryland.

2 teaspoons olive oil	1 teaspoon Worcestershire sauce
½ medium red bell pepper, cut into small dice	1 teaspoon fresh-squeezed lemon juice
⅓ medium yellow bell pepper, cut into small dice	⅛ teaspoon Tabasco sauce, or to taste
¼ medium green bell pepper, cut into small dice	1 pound lump or backfin crabmeat, picked through
¼ cup minced scallions, green and white parts	1 cup all-purpose flour
1 tablespoon chopped fresh parsley	1 large egg
Salt and fresh-ground black pepper	3 large egg whites
½ cup low-fat mayonnaise (1 fat gram per tablespoon)	2 cups fine fresh bread crumbs (from about 4 slices)
½ cup coarse fresh bread crumbs (from about 1 slice)	Lemon wedges
1 large egg	Honey Mustard Sauce (page 130)
2 teaspoons Dijon mustard	

1. Place a nonstick skillet over medium heat and add the oil. When it is hot, add the bell peppers, scallions and parsley and cook, stirring frequently, for 5 to 6 minutes, or until softened; do not brown. Season to taste with salt and pepper and set aside to cool.

2. In a large mixing bowl, whisk together the mayonnaise, coarse bread crumbs, egg, mustard, Worcestershire sauce, lemon juice and Tabasco sauce. Stir in the crabmeat and cooled vegetables.

3. Place the broiler rack 6 inches from the heat source and preheat the broiler. Lightly spray a broiler pan with butter-flavored vegetable oil. Set aside.

4. Put 2 pieces of wax paper on the counter, with a small bowl between them. Put the flour on the first sheet of paper. Put the egg and egg whites in the bowl and whisk until combined. Put the fine bread crumbs on the second sheet of paper.

5. Shape the crab mixture into sixteen 2-inch balls. Coat the balls with the flour, then with the egg mixture, and finally with the bread crumbs. Place on the broiler pan and flatten slightly. Spray the tops of the crab cakes with butter-flavored vegetable oil.

6. Broil the crab cakes for 4 minutes, or until light brown. Turn them over, spray with butter-flavored vegetable oil and broil for 4 minutes more, or until light brown. Serve immediately with the lemon wedges and Honey Mustard Sauce.

Nutritional information per crab cake (without added salt or sauce): 86 calories (24.5% from fat), 2.3 g fat (0.4 g saturated fat), 7.4 g protein, 8.4 g carbohydrate, 43 mg cholesterol, 234 mg sodium.

honey mustard sauce

makes 1¼ cups

My friend Paul, the co-owner of my favorite seafood store in Illinois, graciously shared this recipe with me when I asked him for a good sauce to serve with crab cakes. I substituted low-fat mayonnaise for the high-fat stuff he used, cutting 80 fat grams. Paul's sauce is easy to prepare and tastes terrific with other seafood as well.

- ½ cup prepared yellow mustard
- ½ cup low-fat mayonnaise (1 fat gram per tablespoon)
- ¼ cup clover or other mild honey
- 2 teaspoons minced fresh dill leaves

Place all the ingredients in a small bowl and whisk until combined. Cover and refrigerate for 30 minutes to allow the flavors to blend. Serve chilled.

Nutritional information per tablespoon: 30 calories (25.8% from fat), 0.9 g fat (0 g saturated fat), 0 g protein, 4.9 g carbohydrate, 0 mg cholesterol, 242 mg sodium.

shrimp de jonghe

makes 3 servings as a main course

Shrimp de Jonghe originated as a succulent appetizer served at seafood restaurants on the South Side of Chicago. It usually arrived at the table in a sizzling-hot cast-iron skillet, swimming in a sea of garlic-scented butter. My version has much less butter.

1½ cups fine fresh bread crumbs (from about 4 slices)

2 tablespoons unsalted butter, softened to room temperature

2 tablespoons chopped fresh parsley leaves

3 garlic cloves, crushed and pounded to a paste

1½ pounds large shrimp, shelled and deveined

¼ cup dry sherry (do not use cooking sherry)

Paprika

1. Place the oven rack in the lower-middle position and preheat the oven to 400 degrees. Spray a 9-inch cast-iron skillet with vegetable oil and set aside.

2. Place the bread crumbs, butter, parsley and garlic in a medium mixing bowl. Using your hands, mix until the butter and garlic are evenly distributed.

3. Place the shrimp in a single layer in the skillet, curling them into circles. Pour the sherry over the shrimp. Spoon the crumb mixture evenly over the top, lightly pressing the crumbs onto the shrimp. Sprinkle with the paprika. Bake for 20 minutes, or until the bread crumbs are golden and the shrimp are firm. Serve immediately.

Nutritional information per serving: 394 calories (29% from fat), 12.6 g fat (5.8 g saturated fat), 50.6 g protein, 16.2 g carbohydrate, 370 mg cholesterol, 460 mg sodium.

great grilled spicy shrimp

makes 4 servings

"Great" is no overstatement. Soaking the shrimp in the brine before cooking plumps them up so they are incredibly moist and juicy when they come off the grill. The spicy seasonings are perfect for the sweetness of the shrimp. Purchasing shelled and deveined shrimp makes the preparation of this dish go very quickly.

1 cup kosher salt

2⅓ pounds large shrimp, shelled, leaving the tail and the first shell next to the tail intact, deveined

1 tablespoon chili powder

1½ teaspoons paprika (preferably Hungarian)

1½ teaspoons packed dark brown sugar

1 teaspoon dry ground mustard (preferably Colman's)

Scant 1 teaspoon ground cumin

½ teaspoon fresh-ground black pepper

¼ teaspoon dried oregano, crumbled

¼ teaspoon cayenne pepper

Lemon wedges

1. In a small saucepan, bring 2 cups water to a boil. Place the kosher salt in a large heatproof bowl. Add the boiling water and stir until the salt is mostly dissolved. Add 6 cups ice water (with ice cubes) to the bowl and stir until the salt completely dissolves. Add the shrimp and let stand for 45 minutes.

2. Meanwhile, in a small bowl, stir together the remaining ingredients, except for the lemon wedges. Set aside.

3. Drain and rinse the shrimp thoroughly under cold running water. Arrange them in a single layer on a jelly-roll pan and sprinkle with half the spice mixture. Turn the

shrimp over and sprinkle with the remaining spice mixture. Thread the shrimp onto 4 long metal skewers.

4. Prepare a fire in the grill. When the coals are covered with a light ash, spread them in an even layer. Oil the grill rack, place it 5 to 6 inches over the coals and preheat the rack for 5 minutes.

5. Place the skewers on the grill and cook for 3 minutes. Turn and cook for 3 minutes more, or until the shrimp are pink and offer resistance when pressed. Serve the shrimp immediately on the skewers, with the lemon wedges.

Nutritional information per serving: 258 calories (16% from fat), 4.5 g fat (0.8 g saturated fat), 49 g protein, 4.9 g carbohydrate, 349 mg cholesterol, 566 mg sodium.

cookingtip: If you are going to serve the shrimp cold, make sure to coat them with as much of the spice mixture as possible, since chilling dulls the flavor.

leansuggestion: Serve with spring peas and sliced ripe tomatoes. I ask my guests to shell the peas. A margarita made with good tequila doesn't hurt, either.

citrus-cilantro shrimp

makes about 24 shrimp, or 3 servings as a main course

When a friend shared this recipe with me, I was skeptical. Orange marmalade and shrimp didn't sound like a great combination, but I tried it anyhow, using the best orange marmalade I could buy. When I brought the shrimp out before dinner, one guest exclaimed, "These are great — sweet and hot, absolutely sensational!" I agree.

½ cup fresh-squeezed lime juice

¼ cup orange marmalade

¼ cup fine-chopped cilantro

3 tablespoons slightly thickened chicken broth (page 240)

3 large garlic cloves, minced and pounded to a paste with 1 teaspoon salt

1 tablespoon reduced-sodium soy sauce

½ teaspoon cayenne pepper, or to taste

1½ pounds large shrimp, shelled (leaving tail and first shell next to the tail intact), deveined

1 tablespoon olive oil, *divided*

Fresh cilantro sprigs

1. Whisk together the lime juice, marmalade, cilantro, broth, garlic paste, soy sauce and cayenne in a small bowl. Place two-thirds of the mixture into a large recloseable plastic bag, add the shrimp and press out as much air as possible. Seal the bag, shake it to coat the shrimp evenly and marinate in the refrigerator for 45 minutes. Reserve the remaining one-third of the mixture.

2. Place the oven rack in the lower-middle position and preheat the oven to 170 degrees. Place an ovenproof plate in the oven.

3. Drain the shrimp and lightly pat dry between paper towels; discard the marinade. Place a large nonstick skillet over medium-high heat and add 1½ teaspoons of the oil. When it is hot, add half the shrimp and cook, stirring, until lightly browned and

cooked through, about 1½ minutes on each side. Transfer the cooked shrimp to the plate in the oven. Repeat, cooking the remaining shrimp in the remaining 1½ teaspoons oil.

4. Place the second batch of shrimp on the warm plate and garnish with the cilantro sprigs. Place the reserved marmalade mixture in the center of the plate for dipping and serve immediately.

Nutritional information per shrimp: 43 calories (21% from fat), 0.9 g fat (0.2 g saturated fat), 5.4 g protein, 3.3 g carbohydrate, 37 mg cholesterol, 168 mg sodium.
As a main course: 340 calories (21% from fat), 7.9 g fat (1.3 g saturated fat), 43 g protein, 26.5 g carbohydrate, 296 mg cholesterol, 1,300 mg sodium.

saltsense: Omitting the teaspoon of salt mashed with the garlic reduces the sodium per main-course serving to 636 mg.

cookingtip: A nonstick skillet is an absolute necessity for this dish. I once cooked the shrimp in a cast-iron skillet and spent a lot of time scraping the caramelized marmalade off the bottom.

north carolina shrimp pilaf

makes 6 servings

Pilafs are a delectable mixture of rice, spices, vegetables and sometimes fish or poultry. Bacon is always part of an authentic North Carolina pilaf, and bacon grease is commonly used to sauté the vegetables. I use olive oil and add oven-roasted bacon with all the fat trimmed, leaving only the lean and flavorful parts. This pilaf is a meal in itself. Serve it with a green salad and warm bread.

1 tablespoon olive oil
1 small onion, minced
1 green bell pepper, minced
4 medium garlic cloves, minced
1 serrano pepper, minced
2 cups raw long-grain white rice
2 cups fat-free reduced-sodium chicken broth (preferably homemade)
4 thick slices Oven-Roasted Bacon (page 12), lean parts only, crumbled

¾ pound fresh green beans, trimmed and cut into 1-inch pieces
1 pound medium shrimp, peeled, deveined and cut in half
¼ cup red bell pepper, minced
¼ cup fresh cilantro, minced
¾ teaspoon salt
¼ teaspoon fresh-ground black pepper

1. Place a large nonstick skillet over medium-high heat and add the oil. When it is hot, add the onion, green bell pepper, garlic and serrano pepper. Sauté for 5 to 6 minutes, or until the onion is soft. Add the rice to the skillet and sauté for 4 to 5 minutes, or until it is golden. Stir in the broth, 1½ cups water and the bacon and bring to a boil. Cover, reduce the heat to low and simmer for 15 minutes, or until the rice has almost absorbed the liquid.

2. Meanwhile, bring a large pot of water to a boil.

3. Add the green beans to the pot of boiling water and when it returns to a boil, cook, uncovered, for 3 minutes, or until bright green. Drain and set aside.

4. When the rice mixture is done, remove the cover, fluff with a fork and stir in the shrimp and red bell pepper. Cover and cook for 3 minutes, or until the shrimp are pink and offer some resistance when pressed. Stir in the cilantro, salt and pepper. Taste and adjust the seasonings and serve immediately.

Nutritional information per serving: 414 calories (18.2% from fat), 8.4 g fat (2.2 g saturated fat), 23.2 g protein, 61 g carbohydrate, 121 mg cholesterol, 546 mg sodium.

saltsense: Omitting the salt reduces the sodium to 280 mg per serving.

thai shrimp

makes 4 servings

My first experience with Thai food was at a hole-in-the-wall restaurant with Formica table-tops on Chicago's North Side. None of the chairs matched, but the food was exceptional. I had never tasted such an incendiary yet flavorful cuisine. Lime, garlic, ginger and coconut milk exemplify Thai cuisine and are available in most supermarkets.

2 small limes or 1 medium
1 tablespoon canola oil, *divided*
1 small onion, finely chopped
1 garlic clove, minced
1 medium red bell pepper, thinly sliced
2 teaspoons peeled, grated fresh ginger
⅛ teaspoon cayenne pepper (or 1 small fresh cayenne pepper, seeds removed, finely chopped)
¼ pound white button mushrooms, washed, ends trimmed and cut into quarters or thickly sliced
½ teaspoon salt
1 cup light coconut milk (not regular coconut milk or cream of coconut)

½ cup fat-free reduced-sodium chicken broth
1 pound large shrimp, shelled and deveined
2 ounces snow peas, strings removed, cut into matchstick strips
⅓ cup loosely packed fresh cilantro leaves
3 cups hot cooked basmati or jasmine rice (from 1 cup raw rice)

1. With a vegetable peeler, remove six 1-by-¾-inch strips of peel from the lime. Squeeze 2 tablespoons of lime juice. Set aside.

2. Place a 12-inch nonstick skillet over medium heat and add 2 teaspoons of the oil. When it is hot, add the onion and garlic and sauté for 5 minutes, or until tender. Add the bell pepper and cook for 1 minute. Stir in the ginger and cayenne pepper and cook for 1 minute. Transfer the mixture to a small bowl and set aside.

3. Place the skillet over medium-high heat and add the remaining 1 teaspoon oil. When it is hot, add the mushrooms and salt and cook until tender and lightly browned, about 4 minutes. Add the onion mixture, coconut milk, broth, lime peel and juice and bring to a boil. Add the shrimp and cook until they are opaque, 3 to 4 minutes. Stir in the snow peas and cook for 1 minute. Stir in the cilantro. Serve immediately over the rice.

Nutritional information per serving (with rice): 389 calories (25% from fat), 10.8 g fat (3.8 g saturated fat), 27.5 g protein, 42.4 g carbohydrate, 172 mg cholesterol, 495 mg sodium.

cooking**tip**. One cup of light coconut milk has only 12 fat grams (7.5 grams from saturated fat) and no sugar, yet it carries more than enough flavor. In contrast, 1 cup of regular coconut milk has 45 grams of fat (42 grams from saturated fat). Cream of coconut is a different product that is used in desserts and mixed drinks; it has 40 grams of fat per cup (all of them saturated), plus almost 5 ounces of sugar.

pizza, pasta
and comfort casseroles

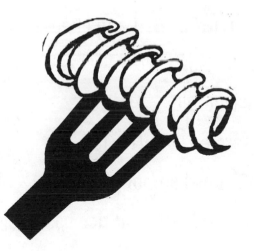

homemade great-eating pizza

plum-good fresh tomato sauce

spaghetti with quick and tasty meat sauce

lickety-split louisiana chicken leanguine

southwestern linguine with shrimp

rotini with peppers, corn and prosciutto

most excellent macaroni and cheese

susan's special lasagna

beefy party casserole

macaroni casserole florentine

potato-crust chicken pot pie

not-your-usual chicken and rice casserole

shrimp and rice dinner casserole

vegetable paella

pizza macaroni casserole

tuna noodle casserole with fresh mushrooms

nawlins-style red beans and rice

black beans and fresh vegetables primavera

hoppin' don

I love casseroles because

they're healthful fast food. On Sunday, I make a casserole that serves eight and refrigerate the leftovers. Then, on Tuesday night, when my wife and I come home late, instead of calling for pizza, I take out two servings and pop them in the microwave. While they are heating, I toss together a salad and dinner is served. No delivery service can ever beat that to the door.

Fast or not, casseroles suffer from a fatty reputation. Traditionally, most of them were made with convenience foods, which cut preparation time but pack in fat and calories. My casseroles and pasta dishes squelch the fat but not the flavor.

Tuna Noodle Casserole with Fresh Mushrooms is a good example. The original recipe came from my grandmother Haynes. Her keys to a great-tasting tuna casserole were canned cream of mushroom soup, oil-packed tuna, real sour cream and potato chips. Instead of canned soup, I added one pound of fresh mushrooms sautéed in a miserly amount of butter and olive oil, then cooked in thickened fat-free chicken broth and skim milk. Switching from oil-packed to water-packed tuna slashed 72 fat grams and 650 unnecessary calories. Substituting nonfat sour cream for the full-fat kind not only lowered the saturated fat and cholesterol but made a smoother sauce. Instead of a topping of potato chips, I used corn flakes. Eggless noodles cut that source of fat to the bone. The result: big servings with only 6 grams of fat.

This chapter is loaded with some of the best dishes I've ever eaten, from Potato-Crust Chicken Pot Pie packed with chicken and vegetables to Susan's Special Lasagna dripping with cheese to Beefy Party Casserole, which fits the bill nicely when you're watching the NBA Finals with the guys.

homemade great-eating pizza

makes 4 to 6 servings

Few pizza joints can equal the pizza I make in my own kitchen. Big plus: I immediately deliver my pizza to the table, hot from the oven, with no waiting for the delivery guy.

What makes my pizza so darned good? First, it bursts with a fine-tuned mixture of flavors. Second, it's lower in calories and fat than any restaurant pizza. Third, there are few things better to help me work out the kinks in my day than banging pizza dough on my kitchen counter when I am kneading it. Finally, I like Italian sausage on my pizza, and the sausage in restaurants is loaded with fat.

sauce

- 1 tablespoon olive oil
- 1 pound All-Beef Italian Sausage (page 76, optional)
- ½ small onion, chopped
- 1 garlic clove, minced
- 1 16-ounce can tomatoes, pureed in a blender
- ¼ cup tomato paste
- 1 teaspoon dried basil, crumbled
- 1 teaspoon dried oregano, crumbled
- ¾ teaspoon salt, or to taste
- ½ teaspoon fresh-ground black pepper
- Pinch of crushed red pepper flakes

dough

- 1 ¼-ounce package Rapid-Rise Yeast
- 1 teaspoon granulated sugar
- 1½ tablespoons olive oil
- 2 garlic cloves, minced
- 3⅓ cups all-purpose flour, *divided*
- ½ teaspoon salt

toppings

- 3 large mushrooms, thinly sliced
- 1 ounce low-fat turkey pepperoni
- 8 ounces low-fat mozzarella cheese, grated (or 4 ounces grated fat-free mozzarella cheese and 4 ounces grated part-skim mozzarella cheese, mixed together)
- 1 medium onion, sliced into paper-thin rings and separated
- 1 red bell pepper, sliced into rings

1. **To make the sauce:** Place a medium saucepan over medium heat and add the oil. When it is hot, add the sausage, if using, and sauté for 2 minutes, breaking it up with the edge of a spoon, until it begins to lose its pink color. Add the onion and garlic and sauté for 3 minutes, or until softened. Stir in ¼ cup water and the remaining ingredients, reduce the heat to low and cook, uncovered, stirring occasionally, for 20 minutes, or until slightly thickened. Cool, transfer to a 1-quart glass jar, seal and refrigerate until needed. (The sauce may be refrigerated for 5 to 7 days or frozen for up to 3 months.)

2. **To make the dough:** Add 1 cup warm (105 to 115 degrees) water to a small bowl; stir in the yeast and sugar. Set aside for 5 minutes, or until foamy.

3. Meanwhile, place a small sauté pan over medium heat and add the oil. When the oil is hot, add the garlic and sauté for 3 minutes, until soft but not brown.

4. Place the garlic-oil mixture, yeast mixture, 3 cups of the flour and the salt in the bowl of a standing mixer fitted with the dough hook. Mix on medium until the dough forms a soft but not sticky ball. If the dough is sticky, add the remaining ⅓ cup flour, 1 tablespoon at a time, mixing it in before adding more. Knead until the dough is very smooth, about 5 minutes.

5. Spray a medium mixing bowl with olive oil. Turn the dough into the bowl. Cover with plastic wrap (do not let it touch the dough) and let rise in a warm area for 40 minutes, or until doubled in bulk.

6. Place the oven rack in the lower-middle position and preheat the oven to 425 degrees. Lightly spray a jelly-roll pan with oil.

7. Turn the dough out into the center of the jelly-roll pan. Using your fingers, press it out until it reaches the edge of the pan.

8. Spread about ⅔ cup of the sauce evenly over the surface of the dough to within ½ inch of the edge. Distribute the mushrooms and pepperoni evenly on the sauce. Sprinkle the cheese over the toppings. Distribute the onion and bell pepper evenly on top of the cheese.

9. Bake for 20 minutes, or until the cheese melts and the crust is golden. Cut the pizza into 16 pieces and serve.

Nutritional information per serving (based on 4 servings): 565 calories (16.5% from fat), 12.7 g fat (4.2 g saturated fat), 28.3 g protein, 82.5 g carbohydrate, 30 mg cholesterol, 1,048 mg sodium.

cookingtip: Don't have a standing mixer? No problem; you can prepare the dough by hand.

Whisk together the garlic-oil and yeast mixtures in a large bowl. Add 3 cups of the flour and the salt. Using a wooden spoon, stir until it becomes difficult to do so. Using clean hands, continue to mix the dough until it forms a soft ball. Sprinkle the counter with flour, place the dough on the flour, dust the top of the dough with additional flour and knead for 5 minutes, or until it is very smooth. (If the dough is sticky, add the reserved flour, 1 tablespoon at a time, kneading it in before adding more.) Proceed as directed in Step 5.

leansuggestion: You can top the pizza in a variety of ways. For suggestions, see page 259.

saltsense: Omitting the salt in the sauce and crust reduces the sodium to 471 mg per serving.

spaghetti with plum-good fresh tomato sauce

makes 2 servings

Choose fresh, ripe plum tomatoes for this sauce because they are meaty and contribute so much body. Once the sauce is ladled over pasta, the percentage of calories from fat falls below 20. Fresh basil is essential; don't settle for dried.

2½	pounds ripe plum tomatoes, coarsely chopped	¾	cup fresh basil leaves, cut cross-wise into shreds
1	medium onion, finely chopped	2½	teaspoons salt, or to taste, *divided*
3	garlic cloves, left whole, plus 1 garlic clove, minced, *divided*	½	teaspoon granulated sugar
			Pinch of cayenne pepper
1½	tablespoons olive oil	½	pound dried spaghetti

1. Place a 5-quart non-aluminum saucepan over medium heat and add the tomatoes, onion and whole garlic cloves. Bring to a boil, reduce the heat to low, partially cover and simmer for 10 minutes, stirring occasionally, or until the tomatoes disintegrate.

2. Meanwhile, place a small sauté pan over medium heat, add the oil and minced garlic and sauté for 1½ minutes, or until the garlic is fragrant. Set aside.

3. Press the tomato mixture through a food mill with a coarse blade or a sieve to remove most of the seeds and skin. Discard the remaining pulp.

4. Return the tomato puree to the saucepan. Add the garlic-oil mixture and the basil and simmer over low heat for 10 minutes. Stir in 1 teaspoon of the salt, the sugar and cayenne pepper. Taste and adjust the seasonings.

5. Meanwhile, bring 5 quarts water to a rolling boil in a large pot. Stir in the remaining 1½ teaspoons salt. Add the spaghetti and stir until the water returns to a boil. Reduce

the heat slightly and boil for 10 to 12 minutes, or until a strand offers a little resistance when bitten. Drain.

6. Divide the spaghetti between 2 plates. Ladle the sauce over the spaghetti and serve.

Nutritional information per serving: 676 calories (17.3% from fat), 13 g fat (0.9 g saturated fat), 18.6 g protein, 123 g carbohydrate, 0 mg cholesterol, 1,435 mg sodium.

saltsense: Reducing the salt in the sauce to ½ teaspoon and cooking the spaghetti in unsalted water will lower the sodium content to 595 mg per serving.

 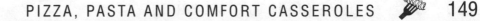

spaghetti with quick and tasty meat sauce

makes 4 servings

When I need dinner in a hurry, this is one recipe I can always turn to, using some of the homemade sausage I keep on hand in the freezer. By the time the pasta is cooked, the sauce is ready.

1½ teaspoons salt
1 pound dried spaghetti
1 tablespoon olive oil
1 cup chopped onion
2 garlic cloves, minced
1 pound All-Beef Italian Sausage (page 76)
1 28-ounce can plum tomatoes, chopped, juice reserved

¼ cup tomato paste
¼ teaspoon crushed red pepper flakes
¼ teaspoon fresh-ground black pepper
1 tablespoon chopped fresh parsley
¼ cup fresh-grated Parmesan cheese

1. Bring 5 quarts water to a rolling boil in a large pot. Stir in the salt. Add the spaghetti and stir until the water returns to a boil. Reduce the heat slightly and boil for 10 to 12 minutes, or until a strand offers a little resistance when bitten. Drain.

2. Meanwhile, place a 5-quart saucepan over medium-high heat and add the oil. When it is hot, add the onion and garlic and cook, stirring, until fragrant, about 2 minutes. Add the sausage and cook, breaking it up with the edge of a spoon, until the meat loses its pink color, 4 to 5 minutes. Add the tomatoes and the reserved juice, reduce the heat to medium and cook, stirring occasionally, until the tomatoes start to disintegrate, about 7 minutes. Stir in the tomato paste, red pepper flakes and black pepper and simmer for 1 minute. Stir in the parsley and simmer for 1 minute more.

3. Divide the spaghetti among 4 plates. Ladle the sauce over the spaghetti. Sprinkle 1 tablespoon cheese on top and serve.

Nutritional information per serving: 699 calories (15.9% from fat), 12.3 g fat (4 g saturated fat), 43 g protein, 102.4 g carbohydrate, 66 mg cholesterol, 1,416 mg sodium.

saltsense: Using no-salt-added tomatoes reduces the sodium to 690 mg per serving. Omitting the salt in the All-Beef Italian Sausage further reduces the sodium to 290 mg per serving.

lickety-split louisiana chicken leanguine

makes 4 servings

I was in a restaurant with my friend Barry when the manager noticed we were both sprinkling crushed red pepper flakes on our bread. He asked if we'd like to taste a piquant dipping
sauce he'd been working on for his new menu. Would we ever! It had a wonderful Louisiana
flavor. After lunch, I returned home to recreate the restaurant's dipping sauce, adding cooked
chicken and serving it over linguine. A great dish was born that night.

1½ teaspoons salt
1 pound dried linguine
2 teaspoons olive oil
1 large red onion, chopped
1 large red bell pepper, chopped
1 large green bell pepper, chopped
½ teaspoon cayenne pepper (or to taste)
1 28-ounce can diced tomatoes with
   their juice

1 cup fat-free reduced-sodium
   chicken broth
2 reduced-sodium chicken bouillon
   cubes
2 teaspoons white vinegar
1 teaspoon dried thyme, crumbled
2 cups cooked, shredded chicken
   breast
2 tablespoons chopped fresh basil

1. Bring 5 quarts water to a rolling boil in a large pot. Stir in the salt. Add the linguine
   and stir until the water returns to a boil. Reduce the heat slightly and boil for 10 to 12
   minutes, or until a strand offers a little resistance when bitten. Drain.

2. Place a 5-quart saucepan over medium-high heat and add the oil. When it is
   hot, add the onion, bell peppers and cayenne and sauté for 5 minutes, or until the
   onion is soft.

3. Add the tomatoes, broth, bouillon cubes, vinegar and thyme, and bring to a boil.
   Reduce the heat to low and simmer for 1 minute, or until the sauce is fragrant.

4. Add the chicken and basil and simmer for 3 minutes more, or until the chicken is heated through and the basil has wilted. Pour the sauce over the linguine, toss to combine and serve.

Nutritional information per serving: 614 calories (8.4% from fat), 5.8 g fat (0.9 g saturated fat), 31.3 g protein, 109.2 g carbohydrate, 37 mg cholesterol, 1,169 mg sodium.

leansuggestion: Shrimp makes a great substitute for the chicken. Add 2 cups cleaned, coarsely chopped raw shrimp along with the basil. Simmer for 3 minutes, or until the shrimp are opaque and offer resistance when pressed with the back of a spoon.

saltsense: Substituting no-salt-added canned tomatoes reduces the sodium per serving to 442 mg.

 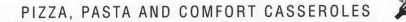

southwestern linguine with shrimp

makes 4 servings

This spectacular dish gets a southwestern spin from spicy jalapeño peppers, tangy lime juice and aromatic fresh cilantro.

2 teaspoons salt, *divided*
½ pound dried linguine
2 tablespoons olive oil, *divided*
½ cup minced onion
6 large garlic cloves, minced
1 pound medium shrimp, shelled and deveined
1 red bell pepper, cut into julienne strips
5 jalapeño peppers, seeded and finely chopped
⅓ cup fine-chopped fresh parsley leaves

¼ cup dry white wine
¼ cup fat-free reduced-sodium chicken broth
2 tablespoons fresh-squeezed lime juice
2 tablespoons fine-chopped fresh cilantro leaves
⅛ teaspoon Tabasco sauce
¼ cup fresh-grated Parmesan cheese

1. Bring 5 quarts water to a rolling boil in a large pot. Stir in 1½ teaspoons of the salt. Add the linguine and stir until the water returns to a boil. Reduce the heat slightly and boil for 10 to 12 minutes, or until a strand offers a little resistance when bitten. Drain.

2. Meanwhile, place a large nonstick skillet over medium heat and add 1 tablespoon of the oil. When the oil is hot, add the onion and garlic and cook, stirring, for 2 minutes, or until beginning to soften. Add the shrimp and cook, stirring, until they are opaque and offer some resistance when pressed with the back of a spoon. With a slotted spoon, transfer them to a large bowl and set aside.

a guy's guide to great eating

3. Add the remaining 1 tablespoon olive oil to the skillet, and when it is hot, add the bell pepper and jalapeño peppers and cook, stirring, until they begin to soften, about 2 minutes. Return the shrimp to the skillet and stir in the parsley, wine, broth, lime juice, cilantro, the remaining ½ teaspoon salt and Tabasco sauce. Add the linguine and toss to coat. Serve immediately with a light sprinkling of Parmesan cheese.

Nutritional information per serving: 452 calories (22.4% from fat), 11.2 g fat (2.4 g saturated fat), 34 g protein, 50.4 g carbohydrate, 179 mg cholesterol, 560 mg sodium.

leansuggestion: This dish is also good with bay scallops substituted for the shrimp. Bay scallops cook very quickly; cook them for 1 minute, or until just opaque.

saltsense: Omitting the salt reduces the sodium to 293 mg per serving.

rotini with peppers, corn and prosciutto

makes 4 servings

This is a flavorful and colorful dinner dish. Since it's made on the stovetop, it's a good choice for a summer evening. Chilled leftovers are terrific for lunch with slices of ripe tomato.

2 teaspoons salt, *divided*
1 pound dried rotini (spiral pasta)
2 teaspoons olive oil
1 medium red onion, finely chopped
1 yellow bell pepper, finely chopped
1 garlic clove, minced
1 cup frozen corn kernels
6 ounces prosciutto or other flavorful ham, trimmed of visible fat and finely chopped
2 7-ounce jars roasted red bell peppers, drained and finely chopped

⅔ cup packed fresh basil leaves, finely chopped
⅔ cup packed fresh parsley leaves, finely chopped
3 tablespoons packed fresh thyme leaves, finely chopped
½ teaspoon fresh-ground black pepper

Lemon wedges
6 tablespoons fresh-grated Parmesan cheese

1. Bring 5 quarts water to a rolling boil in a large pot. Stir in 1½ teaspoons of the salt. Add the rotini and stir until the water returns to a boil. Reduce the heat slightly and boil for 7 to 9 minutes, or until a piece offers a little resistance when bitten. Drain.

2. Meanwhile, place a large nonstick skillet over medium-high heat and add the oil. When it is hot, add the onion, bell pepper and garlic and cook, stirring, until softened, 6 to 7 minutes. Stir in the corn and cook for 2 minutes, or until it begins to

soften. Add the prosciutto or ham and roasted red peppers and cook for 2 minutes, or until heated through.

3. In a large bowl, toss the rotini with the ham mixture, basil, parsley, thyme, the remaining ½ teaspoon salt and pepper. Serve with lemon wedges and pass the Parmesan at the table.

Nutritional information per serving: 681 calories (16.8% from fat), 12.8 g fat (4.3 g saturated fat), 29 g protein, 108.5 g carbohydrates, 44 mg cholesterol, 1,219 mg sodium.

leansuggestion: I serve this with a small platter of ripe tomatoes and warm French bread.

saltsense: Omitting the salt reduces the sodium to 953 mg per serving. Reducing the prosciutto to 3 ounces will further reduce the sodium to 564 mg per serving.

most excellent macaroni and cheese

makes 8 servings, each 1¼ to 1½ cups

Did your mom make macaroni and cheese when you were growing up? Mine did: the best I'd ever tasted. Her secret was Velveeta, an odd "process cheese product" that doesn't need to be refrigerated until it's opened. The downside of her recipe was that 50 percent of its calories came from fat.

Partly inspired by Pam Anderson's *The Perfect Recipe* (1998), which notes that evaporated milk makes a smoother sauce, I created a new version, this time using a combination of evaporated milk, Velveeta Light, reduced-fat cheddar and cottage cheese. This sauce was virtually indistinguishable from my mom's. Once the smoke cleared over my calculator, I found that my new recipe contained even less fat than the previous one. No namby-pamby serving sizes here. Eureka!

2 teaspoons salt, *divided*
1 pound dried macaroni
1 12-ounce can fat-free evaporated milk
½ cup 1% milk
1½ teaspoons dry mustard (preferably Colman's), dissolved in 2 teaspoons water
2 tablespoons cornstarch
8 ounces Velveeta Light reduced-fat processed cheese

4 ounces reduced-fat sharp cheddar cheese, grated (about 1 cup grated)
⅓ cup 1% cottage cheese (not Light n' Lively brand)
½ teaspoon fresh-ground black pepper
⅛ teaspoon cayenne pepper
¼ cup nonfat sour cream

1. Bring 5 quarts water to a rolling boil in a large pot. Stir in 1½ teaspoons of the salt. Add the macaroni and stir until the water returns to a boil. Reduce the heat slightly and boil for 8 to 10 minutes, or until a piece offers a little resistance when bitten. Drain and return to the pot.

2. Meanwhile, whisk together the evaporated milk, milk, mustard paste and cornstarch in a medium saucepan. Place the saucepan over medium heat and, stirring, bring almost to a simmer. Add the Velveeta, cheddar and cottage cheese, the remaining ½ teaspoon salt and black and cayenne peppers, and reduce the heat to low. Cook, stirring, until the cheeses melt and the sauce thickens slightly. Stir in the sour cream and remove from the heat.

3. Pour the sauce over the macaroni and cook, stirring, over medium-low heat until heated through, about 1 minute. Serve immediately.

Nutritional information per serving: 381 calories (16.5% from fat), 6.9 g fat (3.7 g saturated fat), 21.8 g protein, 55.5 g carbohydrate, 14 mg cholesterol, 795 mg sodium.

saltsense: Omitting the salt reduces the sodium content to 662 mg per serving.

susan's special lasagna

makes 8 servings

Since it's such a hassle to make lasagna at home, most folks get theirs from the supermarket freezer section or at their favorite Italian restaurant—but at quite a fat price. Using some lean wizardry of her own, my wife surprised me one night by ripping out the high-fat components of regular lasagna, giving the heave-ho to 283 fat grams and over 2,800 calories in the process. My favorite dinner now gets fewer than 20 percent of its calories from fat when accompanied by a green salad with nonfat dressing and some warm Italian bread with no butter.

sauce

- 1 tablespoon olive oil
- 1 small onion, chopped
- 1 garlic clove, minced
- 1 pound 95% lean ground beef
- 2 16-ounce cans plum tomatoes with their juice, pureed in a blender
- 1 6-ounce can tomato paste
- ½ teaspoon dried basil, crumbled (or 1 tablespoon chopped fresh basil leaves)
- ⅛ teaspoon fresh-ground black pepper

lasagna

- 1 cup fresh-grated Romano or Parmesan cheese, *divided*
- 12 ounces dried lasagna noodles, uncooked, *divided*
- 2 cups 1% cottage cheese, drained (or 16 ounces reduced-fat ricotta cheese), *divided*
- 16 ounces reduced-fat mozzarella cheese (3 fat grams per ounce), grated, *divided*

1. **To make the sauce:** Place a 5-quart saucepan over medium heat and add the oil. When it is hot, add the onion and garlic and sauté for 3 minutes, or until softened. Add the ground beef and cook for 5 minutes, breaking it up with the edge of a spoon, until it loses its pink color. Stir in 2 cups water and the remaining ingredients. Reduce the heat to low and simmer for 1 hour, stirring occasionally. Set aside. (The sauce may be prepared in advance and refrigerated.)

2. Place the oven rack in the center position and preheat the oven to 350 degrees.

3. **To make the lasagna:** Spread one-quarter of the sauce in the bottom of an 11-by-9-by-3-inch baking dish. Sprinkle with one-quarter of the Romano or Parmesan cheese. Place four of the uncooked noodles over the cheese (do not overlap; give them room to expand). Spread one-third of the cottage cheese or ricotta and one-third of the mozzarella cheese over the noodles. Repeat the layers two more times, ending with the remaining sauce and Romano or Parmesan cheese. Cover with foil and bake for 45 minutes. Remove the foil and bake for 15 minutes more, or until the pasta is soft and the top is lightly browned. Serve immediately.

Nutritional information per serving: 480 calories (29.9% from fat), 15.9 g fat (3.9 g saturated fat), 40.2 g protein, 45 g carbohydrate, 104 mg cholesterol, 1,236 mg sodium.

cooking**tips**: In this recipe, the noodles do not need to be cooked, drained and cooled before assembling the lasagna. Use uncooked regular lasagna noodles; they will absorb the sauce and cook in the oven. Do not use "no boil" noodles.

◆ If there is any liquid on the surface of the ricotta, pour it off before spreading it on the lasagna.

saltsense: Using no-salt-added tomatoes reduces the sodium to 841 mg per serving.

beefy party casserole

makes 6 servings

When I have a bunch of guys over to watch a basketball game on TV, I don't want to serve them salty, high-fat snacks. I throw this casserole together just before everyone arrives. While we're having some beers during the pregame show, it bubbles away in my oven.

1½ teaspoons salt
½ pound dried wide yolkless egg noodles
1 teaspoon olive oil
1½ pounds 93%–95% lean ground beef
⅓ cup chopped onion
1 teaspoon Worcestershire sauce
1 teaspoon fresh-ground black pepper
1 teaspoon dried basil, crumbled

1 teaspoon dried marjoram, crumbled
3 8-ounce cans tomato sauce
8 ounces fat-free cream cheese, at room temperature
1 cup 1% cottage cheese
¼ cup nonfat sour cream
⅓ cup chopped green olives

1. Bring 5 quarts water to a rolling boil in a large pot. Stir in the salt. Add the noodles and stir until the water returns to a boil. Reduce the heat slightly and boil for 10 to 12 minutes, or until a noodle offers a little resistance when bitten. Drain and set aside.

2. Place the oven rack in the center and preheat the oven to 350 degrees. Spray a large baking dish with vegetable oil and set aside.

3. Meanwhile, place a large nonstick skillet over medium-high heat and add the oil. When it is hot, add the ground beef and onion and cook, breaking up the meat with the edge of a spoon, until it loses its pink color, 5 to 6 minutes. Add the Worcestershire sauce, pepper, basil and marjoram and cook for 1 minute, or until fragrant. Add the tomato sauce, reduce the heat to medium-low and simmer for 5 minutes.

 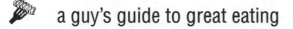

4. Place the cream cheese, cottage cheese and sour cream in a large mixing bowl and mix with an electric mixer on medium until combined, about 2 minutes. Stir in the olives by hand. Set aside.

5. Place half the cooked noodles in the bottom of the casserole and spoon the cheese mixture over them. Evenly distribute the remaining noodles over the cheese. Spoon the beef mixture over the noodles. Bake for 40 to 45 minutes, or until the casserole is bubbling. Serve hot.

Nutritional information per serving: 436 calories (20% from fat), 9.7 g fat (2.9 g saturated fat), 44.7 g protein, 41.1 g carbohydrate, 108 mg cholesterol, 1,361 mg sodium.

saltsense: Substituting no-salt-added tomato sauce for regular will reduce the sodium per serving to 623 mg.

macaroni casserole florentine

makes 6 servings

Spinach is one of my favorite vegetables. There is something about its earthy flavor that makes my mouth water. Fresh spinach is the best, but frozen is a good alternative. I hate . . . hate . . . hate . . . canned spinach.

Whenever I get a hankering for spinach, I put together this casserole.

1½ teaspoons salt
½ pound dried macaroni
½ pound 93%–95% lean ground beef
1 cup fine-chopped onion
1 garlic clove, minced
1 28-ounce can tomato sauce
½ teaspoon dried basil, crumbled
½ teaspoon dried oregano, crumbled
1 10-ounce package frozen chopped spinach, thawed

2 cups 1% cottage cheese
½ cup fresh-grated Parmesan cheese
2 large egg whites, beaten
¼ teaspoon fresh-ground black pepper
4 ounces reduced-fat sharp cheddar cheese, diced, *divided*

1. Place the oven rack in the center and preheat the oven to 375 degrees. Lightly spray a 2-quart baking dish with vegetable oil.

2. Bring 5 quarts water to a rolling boil in a large pot. Stir in the salt. Add the macaroni and stir until the water returns to a boil. Reduce the heat slightly and boil for 7 to 9 minutes, or until a piece offers a little resistance when bitten. Drain and set aside.

3. Meanwhile, place the ground beef, onion and garlic in a large nonstick skillet and sauté over medium-high heat until the meat loses its pink color and the onions are

soft, 5 to 6 minutes. Add the tomato sauce, basil and oregano, reduce the heat and simmer for 5 minutes.

4. Place the spinach in a large strainer in the sink and press out the water with the back of a spoon until very dry. In a medium bowl, stir together the spinach, cottage cheese, Parmesan cheese, egg whites and pepper. Set aside.

5. Spread half the macaroni in the bottom of the baking dish, distribute half the cheddar over the macaroni and then half the meat sauce. Cover the meat sauce with all the spinach mixture. Spread the remaining macaroni over the spinach mixture, then the remaining cheese, and end with the remaining meat sauce. Bake for 35 to 40 minutes, or until the casserole is bubbling around the edges. Serve.

Nutritional information per serving: 392 calories (20.3% from fat), 8.8 g fat (4.5 g saturated fat), 26 g protein, 45.3 g carbohydrate, 29 mg cholesterol, 1,429 mg sodium.

saltsense: Most of the sodium comes from the tomato sauce. Substituting no-salt-added tomato sauce will reduce the sodium per serving to 659 mg.

potato-crust chicken pot pie

makes 6 servings

This recipe takes more than a little effort, but it will be the best pot pie you ever tasted. I guarantee it. And you don't have to make pie crust or biscuits.

2 pounds boneless, skinless chicken breasts

3 cups fat-free reduced-sodium chicken broth

1 tablespoon olive oil

1 large onion, finely chopped

3 medium carrots, peeled and cut into ¼-inch-thick rounds

2 celery ribs, strings removed and cut into ¼-inch-thick pieces

¾ cup frozen baby peas, thawed

¼ cup minced fresh parsley leaves

2 tablespoons butter

2 tablespoons all-purpose flour

½ cup skim milk

½ teaspoon dried thyme, crumbled

3 tablespoons dry sherry (not cooking sherry)

½ teaspoon salt

½ teaspoon fresh-ground black pepper
Seemingly Sinful Fat-Free Roasted Garlic Whipped Potatoes (page 190), prepared with a little extra milk so they are spreadable

Paprika

1. Place the oven rack in the lower-middle position and preheat the oven to 400 degrees. Spray a 13-by-9-inch baking dish with vegetable oil and set aside.

2. Place the chicken breasts and broth in a 4-quart saucepan, cover and bring to a simmer over medium heat. Simmer, stirring occasionally, for 8 to 10 minutes, or until the chicken is cooked through. Transfer to a large bowl and set aside to cool slightly. Measure 2 cups of the broth and set aside; discard the remaining broth.

 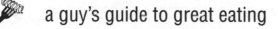

3. Place a medium saucepan over medium-high heat and add the oil. When it is hot, add the cooked onion, carrots and celery and sauté for 5 minutes, or until tender.

4. Tear the chicken into shreds. Stir in the onion mixture, peas and parsley and set aside.

5. Place a medium saucepan over medium heat and add the butter. When it begins to foam, add the flour and cook, stirring, for 3 to 4 minutes, or until it begins to brown. Stir in the reserved broth, milk and thyme, scraping up any browned bits on the bottom of the pan. Bring to a simmer and cook, stirring, until thickened, about 1 minute. Stir in the sherry, salt and pepper.

6. Pour the sauce over the chicken mixture and stir until combined. Taste and adjust the seasonings. Pour the chicken mixture into the prepared baking dish. Spread the whipped potatoes over the top and sprinkle generously with paprika. Bake for 30 minutes, or until the potatoes are golden brown and the filling is bubbly. Serve immediately.

Nutritional information per serving: 464 calories (17.7% from fat), 9.1 g fat (3.7 g saturated fat), 43.1 g protein, 47.9 g carbohydrate, 101 mg cholesterol, 744 mg sodium.

cookingtip: If you are handy with a pastry bag, the whipped potatoes can be piped back and forth over the chicken mixture using a star tip.

leansuggestion: A green salad with your favorite low-fat or nonfat dressing is all you will need to complete this meal.

saltsense: Omitting the salt in the whipped potatoes and in the filling will reduce the sodium to 373 mg per serving. Using no-salt-added chicken broth will further reduce it to 241 mg per serving.

not-your-usual chicken and rice casserole

makes 6 servings

My chicken and rice casserole is much fresher and bolder-tasting than the traditional canned-soup-based version. It starts with chicken breasts marinated in lemon juice and oregano. The rice is seasoned with onion, garlic and ginger. Carrots and peas add color and more flavor.

¼ cup fresh-squeezed lemon juice

1 teaspoon dried oregano, crumbled

½ teaspoon salt

½ teaspoon fresh-ground black pepper

6 skinless bone-in chicken breast halves (about 3 pounds)

3 cups basmati rice

2 tablespoons olive oil

1 large onion, halved lengthwise and thinly sliced crosswise

2 large garlic cloves, minced

1 teaspoon peeled, fine-grated fresh ginger

½ teaspoon paprika

4 cups fat-free reduced-sodium chicken broth

2 medium carrots, peeled and diced

½ teaspoon salt

1 10-ounce package frozen baby peas

1. In a small bowl, whisk together the lemon juice, oregano, salt and pepper.

2. Cut 2 parallel diagonal slits in the thickest part of each chicken breast, cutting down to the bone but being careful not to cut through the edge. Place the chicken in a recloseable plastic bag and add the lemon mixture. Press out as much air as possible, seal and shake the bag to coat the chicken. Let marinate at room temperature for 30 minutes.

3. Meanwhile, rinse the rice in a large bowl, using several changes of cold water, until the water runs clear. Cover the rice with water and let soak for 30 minutes. Drain and set aside.

4. Place the oven rack in the lower-middle position and preheat the oven to 350 degrees.

5. Place a large Dutch oven over medium-high heat and add the oil. When it is hot, add the onion and sauté until golden, about 8 minutes. Add the garlic and sauté for 10 seconds, or until fragrant. Stir in the ginger and sauté for 5 seconds, or until fragrant. Add the chicken, reserving the marinade, and sauté, turning once, for 4 minutes, or until just starting to color. Reduce the heat to medium, add the paprika and stir for 30 seconds. Add the rice and cook, stirring, for 2 minutes. Add the broth, carrots, the reserved marinade and salt. Bring to a boil, cover and place in the oven.

6. Bake for 30 minutes. Stir in the peas, cover and bake for 5 minutes more, or until the rice has absorbed all the liquid. Serve hot.

Nutritional information per serving: 603 calories (12.3% from fat), 8.3 g fat (1.6 g saturated fat), 37.3 g protein, 88.7 g carbohydrate, 73 mg cholesterol, 750 mg sodium.

cookingtip: Basmati rice, an aromatic rice used in Indian cuisine, has a terrific flavor and aroma and can usually be found in the supermarket rice section. Texmati rice, which is grown in Texas, has a wide distribution in supermarkets and can be substituted for basmati. You can also use long-grain white rice; omit step 3.

saltsense: Omitting the salt reduces the sodium to 396 mg per serving. Using no-salt-added chicken broth further reduces it to 146 mg per serving.

shrimp and rice dinner casserole

makes 4 servings

The letter began: "I make this shrimp dish for company, and I always give out the recipe before the night is through. But I'm afraid to think about what the fat and calorie content really is, and I would really appreciate some help . . ."

I would have been afraid to look closely, too. Each serving had 550 calories—not terribly bad—but the fat . . . geeeesh: 35 fat grams per serving with almost 60 percent of the calories coming from fat.

By cutting the oil and the butter, substituting nonfat sour cream diluted with a little skim milk for the whipping cream and reducing the amount of almonds in the topping, I gave my correspondent a dish he could proudly serve.

shrimp
1½ pounds medium raw shrimp, peeled and deveined
1 tablespoon fresh-squeezed lemon juice
1 tablespoon olive oil

casserole
1 teaspoon olive oil
¼ cup minced green bell pepper
¼ cup minced onion
1 (10¾ ounces) can Campbell's Healthy Request condensed tomato soup, undiluted
1 cup nonfat sour cream
2 tablespoons skim milk

rice
1½ cups fat-free reduced-sodium chicken broth (preferably homemade)
¾ cup long-grain white rice

4–6 drops almond extract
1 teaspoon salt
⅛ teaspoon fresh-ground black pepper
⅛ teaspoon ground mace
Cayenne pepper, to taste
2 tablespoons fine-chopped almonds
Paprika to taste

1. **To make the shrimp:** Bring a large saucepan of salted water to a boil, add the shrimp and cook for 3 minutes, or until opaque. Drain. Place the shrimp in a 2-quart baking dish. Sprinkle the lemon juice and oil over the shrimp. Cover and refrigerate for 1 hour.

2. **To make the rice:** Place the broth and rice in a small saucepan and bring to a boil over high heat. Reduce the heat to low and simmer for 18 minutes, or until the broth is absorbed. Remove from the heat and let stand, covered, for 5 minutes. Cool to room temperature.

3. Place the oven rack in the lower-middle position and preheat the oven to 350 degrees.

4. **To make the casserole:** Place a large nonstick skillet over medium heat and add the oil. When it is hot, add the bell pepper and onion and sauté for 4 to 5 minutes, or until soft. Add the cooked rice, onion mixture, tomato soup, sour cream, skim milk, almond extract, salt, pepper, mace and cayenne to the baking dish with the shrimp; mix well. Top with the almonds and paprika. Bake, uncovered, for 55 minutes, or until bubbling. Serve hot.

Nutritional information per serving: 510 calories (19.2% from fat), 11 g fat (1.8 g saturated fat), 45 g protein, 57 g carbohydrate, 266 mg cholesterol, 1,145 mg sodium.

saltsense: Omitting the salt reduces the sodium per serving to 612 mg.

vegetable paella

makes 6 servings

Paella is a Spanish dish. It has three basic ingredients: rice, saffron (the expensive but flavorful red stigmas from the saffron crocus) and olive oil. Make this nontraditional paella in late summer when fresh, ripe tomatoes and Swiss chard are still available.

¼ teaspoon saffron threads

1 tablespoon olive oil

1 red bell pepper, diced

1 medium onion, diced

1 cup skinned, seeded and chopped plum tomatoes

½ 9-ounce package frozen baby artichokes, thawed and quartered

2 large garlic cloves, minced

1½ cups medium-grain white rice

3 cups fat-free reduced-sodium vegetable broth

2 cups chopped Swiss chard leaves

¾ teaspoon paprika

½ teaspoon salt

½ teaspoon fresh-ground black pepper

⅛ teaspoon cayenne pepper, or to taste

1 15-ounce can red kidney beans, drained

½ cup frozen baby peas, thawed

1. Bring ½ cup water to a boil in a small saucepan. Remove from the heat, add the saffron and let stand for 10 minutes.

2. Meanwhile, place a 5-quart nonstick saucepan over medium-high heat and add the oil. When it is hot, add the bell pepper and onion and sauté for 8 minutes, or until golden. Add the tomatoes, artichokes and garlic and sauté for 5 minutes, or until the tomatoes soften. Add the rice and stir to coat. Add the broth and Swiss chard and bring to a boil, stirring frequently so the rice does not stick. Add the saffron water,

 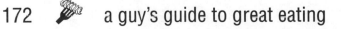

paprika, salt, and black and cayenne peppers. Reduce the heat to low, cover and simmer for 15 minutes. Stir in the beans, cover and simmer for 5 minutes, or until heated through. Remove from the heat, stir in the peas, cover and let stand for 5 minutes, or until the peas are hot. Serve.

Nutritional information per serving: 328 calories (8.2% from fat), 3 g fat (0.5 g saturated fat), 12.5 g protein, 64 g carbohydrate, 0 mg cholesterol, 441 mg sodium.

leansuggestions: You can substitute 2 cups fresh spinach leaves, stems removed, for the Swiss chard.

- ◆ Substitute a 10-ounce package of frozen chopped spinach, defrosted and squeezed dry, for the Swiss chard. Add with the kidney beans.

pizza macaroni casserole

makes 8 servings

Part pizza, part casserole, this dish delivers less than 7 fat grams per serving. It's even better reheated the next day.

1½ teaspoons salt
½ pound dried macaroni
½ cup skim milk
1 large egg
1½ cups fat-free spaghetti sauce
1 15-ounce can kidney beans, drained
7 ounces low-fat smoked sausage, such as kielbasa, thinly sliced
1 small green bell pepper, diced
1 small tomato, diced
1 small onion, sliced

¼ pound white button mushrooms, cleaned, stems trimmed and thinly sliced
1 2-ounce can chopped mild green chilies, drained
½ teaspoon dried basil, crumbled
½ teaspoon dried oregano, crumbled
2 cups shredded low-fat mozzarella cheese

1. Bring 5 quarts water to a rolling boil in a large pot. Stir in the salt. Add the macaroni and stir until the water returns to a boil. Reduce the heat slightly and boil for 7 to 9 minutes, or until a noodle offers a little resistance when bitten. Drain and set aside.

2. Place the oven rack in the lower-middle position and preheat the oven to 350 degrees. Lightly spray a 13-by-9-inch baking dish with vegetable oil.

3. In a medium mixing bowl, whisk together the milk and egg. Add the cooked macaroni and stir well. Spread the macaroni mixture evenly in the baking dish.

 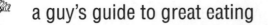

4. Spoon the spaghetti sauce over the macaroni, not quite to the edge. Top with the beans, sausage, bell pepper, tomato, onion, mushrooms and chilies. Sprinkle with the basil and oregano, then distribute the cheese on top. Bake for 30 minutes, or until bubbling. Let stand for 5 minutes before serving.

Nutritional information per serving: 306 calories (20.3% from fat), 6.9 g fat (3.6 g saturated fat), 25 g protein, 39.5 g carbohydrate, 43 mg cholesterol, 593 mg sodium.

cooking**tip**: If you can't find low-fat mozzarella cheese, use 1 cup fat-free mozzarella and 1 cup skim-milk mozzarella.

leansuggestion: If you like smoked sausage, use both links from a 14-ounce package. This addition will increase the calories per serving by 31 and the fat by only 0.7 grams.

 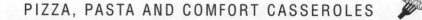

tuna noodle casserole with fresh mushrooms

makes 6 servings

My maternal grandmother, Edna Mae Haynes, made the best tuna casserole in the world. Sour cream made it smooth and richly flavored, and she topped it with crushed potato chips. Here is a much more healthful version of Grandma Haynes' famous tuna casserole for the new millennium.

1½ teaspoons salt
½ pound dried wide yolkless egg noodles
1 tablespoon olive oil
1 tablespoon butter
2 celery ribs, strings removed and chopped
⅓ cup chopped onion
1 garlic clove, minced
1 pound white button mushrooms, cleaned, stems trimmed and sliced
⅓ cup all-purpose flour
3 cups fat-free reduced-sodium chicken broth

1 cup skim milk
½ teaspoon celery salt
½ teaspoon fresh-ground black pepper
2 6½-ounce cans water-packed tuna, drained and broken into flakes
1 cup frozen baby peas
⅓ cup nonfat sour cream
⅓ cup 1% cottage cheese
2 tablespoons chopped fresh parsley

1. Bring 5 quarts water to a rolling boil in a large pot. Stir in the salt. Add the noodles and stir until the water returns to a boil. Reduce the heat slightly and boil for 10 to 12 minutes, or until a noodle offers a little resistance when bitten. Drain and set aside.

2. Place a 5-quart saucepan over medium-high heat and add the oil and butter. When the butter foams, add the celery, onion and garlic and cook, stirring occasionally, until softened, 4 to 5 minutes. Add the mushrooms and cook, stirring occasionally, until

they give off their liquid, about 5 minutes. Stir in the flour and cook until it begins to brown. Stir in the broth, milk, celery salt and pepper, scraping up the browned bits from the bottom of the pan.

3. Add the tuna and stir until combined. Reduce the heat to low, cover and simmer for 5 minutes, stirring occasionally. Add the peas, sour cream and cottage cheese and stir until the cottage cheese curds melt. Stir in the noodles. Cover, remove from the heat and let stand for 5 minutes. Sprinkle the top with the parsley and serve.

Nutritional information per serving: 371 calories (14.3% from fat), 5.9 g fat (1.9 g saturated fat), 30.7 g protein, 47.1 g carbohydrate, 27 mg cholesterol, 713 mg sodium.

saltsense: Using no-salt-added tuna, no-salt-added chicken broth and ½ teaspoon celery seeds instead of celery salt will reduce the sodium to 255 mg per serving.

nawlins-style red beans and rice

makes 6 servings

The traditional recipe for red beans and rice is loaded with fat. I took the traditional seasonings and flavors and created a leaner version without destroying the integrity of the original.

1 tablespoon olive oil
1 large onion, chopped
2 small celery ribs, strings removed and chopped
4 garlic cloves, minced
4 bay leaves
1 tablespoon dried thyme, crumbled
2 teaspoons dried oregano, crumbled
1 teaspoon Tabasco sauce
¾ teaspoon garlic powder
½ teaspoon *each* ground allspice, ground cloves, ground white pepper and fresh-ground black pepper
¼ teaspoon cayenne pepper, or to taste

3 15-ounce cans red kidney beans, including liquid
1 14-ounce package low-fat smoked sausage, halved lengthwise and cut into ¼-inch-thick slices
1 cup fat-free reduced-sodium chicken broth (preferably homemade), plus more if needed

3 cups hot cooked white rice (from 1 cup raw)

1. Place a large nonstick saucepan over medium-high heat and add the oil. When it is hot, add the onion, celery, garlic, bay leaves, thyme, oregano, Tabasco sauce, garlic powder, allspice, cloves and white and black peppers and cayenne. Sauté until the onion is soft, about 5 minutes.

2. Meanwhile, mash 1 cup of the drained kidney beans with a fork and set aside.

3. Add the kidney beans and their liquid, mashed kidney beans, sausage and broth to the saucepan and stir until combined. Reduce the heat to low, cover and simmer, stirring occasionally, for 8 to 10 minutes, or until the sausage is heated through. If the mixture is too thick, thin with more chicken broth. Remove the bay leaves and serve over the prepared rice.

Nutritional information per serving: 511 calories (9.6% from fat), 5.4 g fat (1.3 g saturated fat), 33 g protein, 82 g carbohydrate, 29 mg cholesterol, 961 mg sodium.

saltsense: Using half the sausage reduces the sodium to 682 mg per serving. Progresso red kidney beans are lower in sodium than other brands.

black beans and fresh vegetables primavera

makes 6 servings

In this colorful dish, the black beans deliver an earthy note. The quick-cooked yellow squash, broccoli and green beans add sweetness, and the broccoli contributes crunch.

I serve this primavera with a glass of Beaujolais, a tossed green salad and warm French bread.

beans
- 1 teaspoon olive oil
- 1 small onion, chopped
- 1 garlic clove, minced
- 1 teaspoon ground cumin
- 2 15-ounce cans black beans, drained and rinsed
- ¼ cup fat-free reduced-sodium chicken broth
- ½ teaspoon salt

macaroni
- 2½ cups fat-free reduced-sodium chicken broth
- ½ teaspoon salt
- 5–6 saffron threads
- 1 cup dried macaroni

vegetables
- 1 small yellow summer squash, diced
- 1 cup broccoli florets
- 1 cup diced green beans

garnish
- ½ red bell pepper, thinly sliced
- 6 tablespoons fresh-grated Parmesan cheese

1. **To make the beans:** Place a large nonstick skillet over medium-low heat and add the oil. When it is hot, add the onion, cover and cook until tender, 10 to 12 minutes. Add the garlic and sauté for 2 minutes, or until soft. Add the cumin and cook, stirring, for 30 seconds, or until fragrant. Add the beans, broth and salt and cook until the beans are heated through, 4 to 5 minutes. Cover and keep warm.

2. **To make the macaroni:** Bring the broth to a boil in a 5-quart saucepan. Remove from the heat, stir in the salt and saffron, cover and let stand for 10 minutes. Return to a boil. Add the macaroni, cover and simmer over low heat until it is tender and most of the liquid is absorbed, 8 to 10 minutes.

3. **Meanwhile, make the vegetables:** Bring a large pot of salted water to a boil. Add the squash, broccoli and green beans and cook until crisp-tender, about 3 minutes. Drain.

4. Add the vegetables and beans to the macaroni and stir until combined. Divide the primavera among 6 plates. Garnish with the bell pepper strips, sprinkle with Parmesan cheese and serve.

leansuggestion: You can substitute fat-free reduced-sodium vegetable broth for the chicken broth.

Nutritional information per serving: 213 calories (13.5% from fat), 3.2 g fat (1.2 g saturated fat), 13 g protein, 40.3 g carbohydrates, 4 mg cholesterol, 310 mg sodium.

hoppin' don

makes 8 servings

When I moved to North Carolina, I couldn't turn around without seeing black-eyed peas. In the South, a very special black-eyed pea dish—Hoppin' John—is prepared as part of the New Year's Day meal, to bring good fortune in the new year.

Hoppin' John bursts with flavor. My version of this terrific North Carolina dish has less than 4 fat grams per serving, yet all the good ol' flavor still remains.

8 ounces dried black-eyed peas, sorted and rinsed

1 tablespoon olive oil

1 cup diced onion

2 garlic cloves, minced

½ teaspoon crushed red pepper flakes

1¼ cups raw long-grain white rice

4 cups fat-free reduced-sodium chicken broth

14 ounces low-fat smoked sausage, such as kielbasa, cut crosswise into ½-inch slices

1 bay leaf

1 teaspoon dried thyme, crumbled

⅛ teaspoon ground cloves

½ teaspoon salt, or to taste

¼ teaspoon fresh-ground black pepper

1. In a medium saucepan simmer the black-eyed peas in enough water to cover them by 2 inches for 25 to 30 minutes, or until just tender; drain and set aside.

2. Place the oven rack in the low position and preheat the oven to 325 degrees.

3. Place a Dutch oven over medium heat and add the oil. When it is hot, add the onion, garlic and red pepper flakes. Cook, stirring, until the onions are soft, about 6 minutes.

Add the rice and stir until coated with the oil. Add the broth, sausage, black-eyed peas, bay leaf, thyme and cloves and bring to a boil. Cover and place in the oven. Bake for 20 minutes, or until the rice is tender. Season with the salt and pepper and serve immediately.

Nutritional information per serving: 235 calories (12.8% from fat), 3.3 g fat (0.7 g saturated fat), 13.4 g protein, 31.4 g carbohydrate, 22 mg cholesterol, 757 mg sodium.

saltsense: Omitting the salt reduces the sodium to 623 mg per serving.

 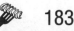

stick to your ribs
sides

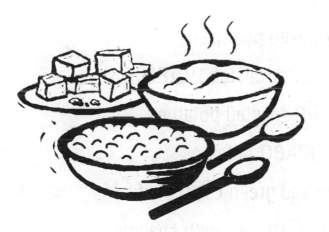

special mashed potatoes

seemingly sinful fat-free
roasted garlic whipped potatoes

easy sweet oven-roasted garlic

steakhouse oven-fried potatoes

boil-n'-bake taters

crispy baked potatoes

southwestern roasted potatoes

aromatic roasted potatoes

twice-baked potatoes

easy rice and green chili pilaf

jazzy jasmine rice with shallots

zesty curried rice pilaf

curried navy beans

fancy sweet corn bread

For satisfaction on a plate, nothing beats a mound of whipped potatoes or an aromatic square of warm corn bread. With side dishes like these, you'll never have to worry about leaving the table hungry.

Unlike traditional versions, these accompaniments don't get their flavor from gobs of butter or sour cream. But I've never met anyone who knew the difference between my Seemingly Sinful Fat-Free Roasted Garlic Whipped Potatoes and the fatty version. Special Mashed Potatoes have uncommon flavor notes and are unbelievably low in fat. They're cooked in a mixture of fat-free chicken broth, white wine and sautéed onions, with finely chopped good-quality black olives stirred in at the end.

Rice can be as satisfying as potatoes, especially if you choose jasmine rice, which is particularly aromatic. When it simmers, it gives off a scent that reminds me of popcorn, and it has a flavor that ordinary white rice can't approach.

Often neglected as a side dish, beans are more filling than potatoes or rice, and their high fiber content makes them powerful cholesterol-fighters. If you can work a can opener, you can serve beans regularly, and they have an unparalleled ability to soak up flavors. In Curried Navy Beans, fresh ginger, hot curry powder and sweet onions prove that the whole can be much more than the sum of its parts.

special mashed potatoes

makes 4 servings

My brother Tom, who is a chef, created these special potatoes. Cooking them in chicken broth and white wine with sautéed onions gives complex flavors to the dish that plain water never could.

1½ teaspoons unsalted butter
½ yellow onion, finely chopped
2 pounds Yukon Gold potatoes, peeled and cut into ¼-inch-thick slices
4 cups fat-free reduced-sodium chicken broth

¼ cup dry white wine
¾ teaspoon salt
¼ teaspoon fresh-ground black pepper
¼ cup kalamata olives, pitted and minced

1. Melt the butter in a 5-quart saucepan over medium heat. Add the onion and sauté until translucent, 3 to 4 minutes; do not let brown. Add the potatoes, broth and wine and bring to a boil. Reduce the heat to low and simmer for 15 to 20 minutes, or until the potatoes can be easily pierced with a knife. Place a colander in a large bowl and pour the potato mixture into the colander; reserve the liquid.

2. Place the potatoes in a large mixing bowl. With an electric mixer on low, begin to break up the potatoes, then increase the speed to medium and mix for 1 to 2 minutes more, until the potatoes start to become smooth. Add ¾ cup of the reserved cooking liquid, salt and pepper and mix until smooth and creamy, about 2 minutes. If the potatoes seem stiff or dry, add up to ¼ cup more cooking liquid.

3. Stir in the olives by hand and serve.

Nutritional information per serving: 245 calories (9.3% from fat), 2.6 g fat (0.9 g saturated fat), 3.8 g protein, 49 g carbohydrate, 4 mg cholesterol, 597 mg sodium.

cooking**tip**: Overmixing the potatoes will make them gummy. So will using a food processor.

saltsense: Omitting the salt will reduce the sodium to 197 mg per serving.

seemingly sinful fat-free roasted garlic whipped potatoes

makes 6 servings

The best potatoes for this dish are russets or Yukon Golds, which have a high starch content. Also, experience has taught me that older potatoes make better whipped potatoes than new ones.

2½ pounds baking (russet) or Yukon Gold potatoes, peeled

¼ cup skim milk, warmed

1 head Easy Sweet Oven-Roasted Garlic (page 192), squeezed out of the cloves

2 tablespoons nonfat sour cream

2 teaspoons Butter Buds, mixed with 2 tablespoons hot water

½ teaspoon salt

¼ teaspoon fresh-ground black pepper

1 tablespoon minced fresh parsley leaves

Paprika to taste

1. Place the potatoes in a 5-quart saucepan and add enough water to cover by 1 inch. Bring to a boil, reduce the heat to medium and simmer for 20 minutes, or until the potatoes can be easily pierced with a knife. Drain.

2. Place the potatoes in a large mixing bowl. With an electric mixer on low, begin to break up the potatoes. As they break up, slowly turn up the speed to medium. Add the milk, roasted garlic, sour cream, Butter Buds, salt and pepper and mix until smooth, about 45 seconds. Taste and adjust the seasonings. Spoon the whipped potatoes into a warmed serving bowl, sprinkle with parsley and paprika and serve.

 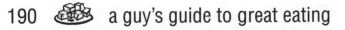

Nutritional information per serving: 170 calories (4.5% from fat), 0.8 g fat (0.4 g saturated fat), 5.5 g protein, 37.5 g carbohydrate, 2.6 mg cholesterol, 212 mg sodium.

leansuggestion: You can also add 1 tablespoon coarse mustard and ½ teaspoon minced fresh tarragon when whipping the potatoes.

easy sweet oven-roasted garlic

Roasted garlic is ambrosial, soft and sweet, with a rounded, mellow flavor. It's better than butter on bread (and almost as spreadable), and can be served as an appetizer. It adds incomparable richness to whipped potatoes.

3 firm heads fresh garlic   1½ teaspoons olive oil, *divided*

1. Place the oven rack in the lower-middle position and preheat the oven to 300 degrees.

2. Lay each garlic head on its side on a cutting board and roll it around, pressing downward to loosen the papery outer skin. Peel away the loose skin. (Stop when it becomes difficult to remove any more.) Cut off about ½ inch from the tip end of each garlic head; discard the tips.

3. Place each garlic head, cut side up, on an 8-inch square of aluminum foil. Drizzle ½ teaspoon of the olive oil over each head. Gather the corners of each square together and twist to seal. Place each packet on the oven rack and roast until very soft, about 1 hour. Let cool.

4. Remove the garlic from the foil and, squeezing from the root end, push the roasted cloves out of the head. The roasted garlic can be mashed with a fork. The puree can be stored, covered, in the refrigerator for up to 1 week.

Nutritional information per garlic head: 67 calories (29.4% from fat), 2.2 g fat (0.3 g saturated fat), trace of protein, 13 g carbohydrate, 0 mg cholesterol, 13 mg sodium.

lean suggestion: Spread roasted garlic on a purchased pizza crust before adding pizza sauce or stir it into Mess o' Mushroom Soup (page 40). Roasted garlic is also what makes my Roasted Garlic Salad Dressing (page 243) so outstanding.

 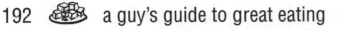

steakhouse oven-fried potatoes

makes 4 servings

These steakhouse-style potatoes are cut in large rectangles and seasoned just right. They emerge from the oven golden brown on the outside and soft and sweet inside. I love to serve them with grilled flank steak and one of my creamy cabbage slaws (pages 226–28).

1½ tablespoons olive oil	4 8-ounce red-skin potatoes,
2 large garlic cloves, minced	scrubbed
1 teaspoon salt	Paprika to taste
½ teaspoon fresh-ground black pepper	

1. Place the oven rack in the lower-middle position and preheat the oven to 425 degrees.

2. Place the oil, garlic, salt and pepper in a large mixing bowl and whisk until combined.

3. Cut the potatoes into finger-size lengths ½ inch thick, 1 inch wide and as long as the potato. Pat the pieces dry with paper towels. Add them to the mixing bowl and toss until coated with oil.

4. Place the potatoes on a jelly-roll pan, making certain they do not touch each other. Sprinkle generously with the paprika. Bake for 15 minutes. Turn the potatoes and sprinkle generously with paprika. Bake for 15 minutes more, or until golden, and serve.

Nutritional information per serving: 229 calories (20.3% from fat), 5.1 g fat (0.7 g saturated fat), 3.8 g protein, 44.1 g carbohydrate, 0 mg cholesterol, 547 mg sodium.

cookingtip: Lining the jelly-roll pan with heavy-duty foil makes for quick and easy cleanup. Omitting the salt reduces the sodium to 14 mg per serving.

boil-n'-bake taters

makes 4 servings

A couple of years after I met Al Carson, a food writer for the *Durham Herald-Sun*, he started to eat healthfully. He sent me the following recipe, writing "Wonderful!" at the end. I couldn't have said it better myself.

2 8-ounce baking (russet) potatoes, cut into 1-inch cubes (peeling is optional)
1 medium onion, coarsely chopped
1 medium green bell pepper, coarsely chopped
2 tablespoons prepared yellow mustard, regular or spicy

2 tablespoons fresh-grated Parmesan cheese
1 teaspoon hot sauce (Al likes Texas Pete, but Tabasco is fine too)
1 teaspoon garlic powder
Nonfat sour cream

1. Place the oven rack in the center and preheat the oven to 300 degrees. Lightly spray a 2-to-3-quart baking dish with vegetable oil and set aside.

2. Fill a 5-quart saucepan two-thirds full of water. Bring to a boil over high heat. Add the potatoes, onion and bell pepper and return to a boil. Reduce the heat slightly and simmer for 15 minutes, or until the potatoes offer a touch of resistance when pierced.

3. In a medium mixing bowl, whisk together the mustard, Parmesan cheese, hot sauce and garlic powder. Drain the potato mixture well, add to the bowl and toss to coat.

4. Place the potato mixture in the baking dish and bake for 30 minutes, or until golden. Serve with the sour cream.

Nutritional information per serving: 123 calories (7.3% from fat), 1.4 g fat (0.5 g saturated fat), 4 g protein, 34.3 g carbohydrate, 2 mg cholesterol, 283 mg sodium.

crispy baked potatoes

makes 4 servings

Oven-browning is an easy way to create a potato with a crisp exterior and soft interior, very much like a French fry. These baked potatoes are as easy as 1-2-3. Cut a slice, drizzle on a little ketchup and chow down.

4 8-ounce baking (russet) potatoes
Salt to taste
2 tablespoons dry bread crumbs

½ teaspoon garlic powder
Paprika to taste

1. Place the oven rack in the center and preheat the oven to 425 degrees. Spray a 13- by 9-inch baking dish with butter-flavored vegetable oil spray and set aside.

2. Peel the potatoes. Trim a thin horizontal slice from each potato so it will remain stable. Make vertical slices in each potato, cutting no more than two-thirds through, about ⅛ inch apart. (Each potato will look like a miniature loaf of bread.) Pat the potatoes dry with a paper towel.

3. Place the potatoes in the baking dish, cut sides up. Spray the tops and sides of each potato with buttered-flavored vegetable oil and sprinkle on a little salt. Bake for 30 minutes. Remove the baking dish from the oven. Spray the potatoes with butter-flavored vegetable oil and sprinkle the bread crumbs, garlic powder and paprika on top. Return to the oven and bake until tender and golden, 25 to 30 minutes more. Serve.

Nutritional information per serving: 274 calories (5.1% from fat), 1.6 g fat (0.2 g saturated fat), 6.3 g protein, 60.4 g carbohydrate, 0 mg cholesterol, 312 mg sodium.

southwestern roasted potatoes

makes 6 servings

With the zing of garlic and cumin, these potatoes go well with grilled burgers or Mahogany Spice-Rubbed Barbecued Turkey (page 114).

1 tablespoon olive oil
1 tablespoon chopped fresh oregano leaves (or 1 teaspoon dried oregano, crushed)
1 tablespoon minced garlic
1 teaspoon chili powder
½ teaspoon ground cumin
½ teaspoon salt
¼ teaspoon fresh-ground black pepper
Cayenne pepper to taste
2 pounds red-skin potatoes (small new potatoes are perfect), scrubbed
Paprika to taste

1. Place the oven rack in the center and preheat the oven to 375 degrees.

2. Place the oil, oregano, garlic, chili powder, cumin, salt, pepper and cayenne in a large mixing bowl and stir until combined. Set aside.

3. If using large potatoes, cut them into 1-inch chunks; leave small new potatoes whole. Pat dry with paper towels.

4. Add the potatoes to the mixing bowl and toss to coat. Place the potatoes in a single layer in a jelly-roll pan. Sprinkle with the paprika. Bake for 45 to 60 minutes, stirring every 15 minutes, or until golden brown. Serve hot.

Nutritional information per serving: 142 calories (16% from fat), 2.6 g fat (0.3 g saturated fat), 4 g protein, 28 g carbohydrate, 0 mg cholesterol, 193 mg sodium.

aromatic roasted potatoes

makes 4 servings

I sauté these potatoes on top of the stove before they go into the oven and season them with oregano, parsley, garlic and wine. They're delicious with grilled chicken breasts.

½ cup fresh parsley leaves
4 large garlic cloves
2 teaspoons dried oregano, crumbled
1½ tablespoons olive oil
6 medium baking (russet) potatoes, peeled, halved crosswise, each half quartered lengthwise

3 tablespoons dry white wine
Salt and fresh-ground black pepper

1. Place the oven rack in the center and preheat the oven to 425 degrees.

2. Place the parsley, garlic and oregano in a food processor with the steel blade in place and process until finely minced, about 5 seconds. Set aside.

3. Place a large ovenproof skillet over medium-high heat and add the oil. When it is hot, add the potatoes in a single layer and cook until just starting to brown, 2 to 3 minutes per side.

4. Transfer the skillet to the oven and bake for 20 minutes. Turn the potatoes, sprinkle with the garlic mixture and wine and toss to combine. Season with salt and pepper to taste. Bake for 10 minutes more, or until the potatoes can be easily pierced with a knife. Transfer to a warm platter and serve.

Nutritional information per serving (without added salt): 207 calories (23.1% from fat), 5.3 g fat (0.8 g saturated fat), 3.3 g protein, 36.9 g carbohydrate, 0 mg cholesterol, 17 mg sodium.

twice-baked potatoes

makes 4 servings

Twice-baked potatoes are twice as good as ordinary baked potatoes — and twice as high in fat, thanks to butter, cream, sour cream and cheese. These potatoes are just twice as high in flavor.

4　8-ounce baking (russet) potatoes, scrubbed and pierced in 2 or 3 places with a knife

4　tablespoons reduced-fat soft tub margarine (2 fat grams per tablespoon)

½　teaspoon salt

¼　teaspoon fresh-ground black pepper

½　cup nonfat sour cream

½　cup fresh-grated Parmesan cheese, *divided*

1　large egg yolk
　Paprika to taste

1. Place the oven rack in the center and preheat the oven to 425 degrees.

2. Bake the potatoes for 55 to 60 minutes, or until tender and cooked through.

3. Holding each potato with an oven mitt, remove the tops by slicing lengthwise. With a spoon, scoop out the potato flesh and place in a mixing bowl; reserve the skins. Add the margarine, salt and pepper to the bowl and break up the potatoes with an electric mixer on low. Turn up the mixer to medium and mix until coarse.

4. Add the sour cream and ¼ cup of the Parmesan cheese and mix until smooth. Add the egg yolk and mix until blended.

5. Spoon the mixture into the potato skins, sprinkle with the remaining ¼ cup Parmesan cheese and the paprika. Place the potatoes on a jelly-roll pan and bake for 7 to 10 minutes, or until heated through and lightly browned. Serve immediately.

Nutritional information per serving: 337 calories (17.3% from fat), 6.5 g fat (2.6 g saturated fat), 11.8 g protein, 57.6 g carbohydrate, 66 mg cholesterol, 603 mg sodium.

saltsense: Omitting the salt reduces the sodium to 337 mg per serving.

 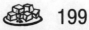

easy rice and green chili pilaf

makes 4 servings

Chop a little onion and garlic and toss it into a skillet with diced chilies, add some chicken broth and rice, and in 20 minutes you'll have a terrific-tasting, fluffy rice pilaf on the table.

2 teaspoons olive oil	1½ cups fat-free reduced-sodium chicken broth (preferably homemade)
1 medium onion, finely chopped	
1 cup white basmati rice	¼ teaspoon salt
2 4-ounce cans chopped mild green chilies, drained	¼ teaspoon fresh-ground black pepper
2 large garlic cloves, minced	2 scallions, green parts only, thinly sliced

Place a heavy nonstick saucepan over medium-low heat and add the oil. When it is hot, add the onion and cook, stirring, for 5 minutes, or until softened. Stir in the rice, chilies and garlic and cook, stirring, until the rice is translucent, about 1 minute. Add the broth, salt and pepper and bring to a boil. Reduce the heat to low and cook, covered, until the liquid is absorbed and the rice is tender, about 20 minutes. Fluff with a fork, stir in the scallions and serve.

Nutritional information per serving: 214 calories (10.6% from fat), 2.5 g fat (0.4 g saturated fat), 4 g protein, 42.7 g carbohydrate, 0 mg cholesterol, 358 mg sodium.

cookingtip: Basmati rice, an aromatic rice with a wonderful aroma and flavor, can be found in the rice section of most supermarkets. Texmati rice, a basmati grown in Texas, or long-grain white rice can be substituted.

saltsense: Omitting the salt reduces the sodium to 225 mg per serving.

jazzy jasmine rice with shallots

makes 4 servings

This is a perfect accompaniment to main-course dishes calling for rice. Jasmine rice has a wonderful aroma and a great flavor. The shallots add their own sweet garlicky notes, while the chicken broth enriches everything.

2　teaspoons olive or toasted sesame oil
1　small shallot, peeled and thinly sliced
1　cup long-grain jasmine rice

1　cup fat-free reduced-sodium chicken broth

1. Place a small nonstick saucepan over medium-high heat and add the oil. When it is hot, add the shallot and sauté until soft, about 2 minutes. Add the rice and stir to coat with the oil.

2. Add the broth and ⅔ cup water to the saucepan and bring to a boil. Reduce the heat to low, cover and simmer gently for 18 minutes (do not remove cover). Remove from the heat and let stand for 5 minutes. Fluff with a fork and serve.

Nutritional information per serving: 197 calories (11.3% from fat), 2.5 g fat (0.4 g saturated fat), 3.5 g protein, 39 g carbohydrate, 0 mg cholesterol, 102 mg sodium.

cooking**tip**: Jasmine rice is of East Asian origin, and you've probably tasted it at your favorite Chinese or Thai restaurant. It is available in a domestic version at many supermarkets as Jasmati. Jasmine rice may also be found at health or natural food stores as well as East Asian markets.

zesty curried rice pilaf

makes 6 servings

Thanks to the curry powder, this pilaf has such a stand-out flavor that I serve it with meats that are not highly seasoned, such as roast beef or turkey breast. A slightly sweet vegetable, such as steamed peas or carrots, goes well with it. The spiciness of curry powder is determined by the amount of hot pepper it contains. I keep several different brands on my spice rack.

1½ cups basmati rice (see tip, page 200)
1 tablespoon butter
1 medium onion, chopped
1 tablespoon hot curry powder
⅛ teaspoon cayenne pepper

2½ cups fat-free reduced-sodium chicken broth (preferably homemade)
½ teaspoon salt
3 tablespoons chopped fresh parsley leaves

1. Place the rice in a medium bowl and cover with cold water. Stir the water around to remove the starch coating on the rice. Drain and continue washing and draining until the water is clear. Add enough warm water to cover the rice by 1 inch. Soak for 20 minutes. Drain.

2. After the rice has soaked for 15 minutes, place a medium nonstick saucepan over medium heat and add the butter. When it foams, add the onion and cook, stirring, for 5 minutes, or until softened. Add the drained rice and stir until coated with butter. Add the curry powder and cayenne pepper and cook, stirring, for 1 minute, or until fragrant.

3. Add the broth and salt to the saucepan and bring to a boil. Reduce the heat to low, cover and simmer until the rice is tender and the liquid is absorbed, about 17 minutes.

4. Remove from the heat and let stand, covered, for 5 minutes. Add the parsley and fluff the rice with a fork. Serve.

Nutritional information per serving: 204 calories (10.5% from fat), 2.4 g fat (1.9 g saturated fat), 4 g protein, 40.8 g carbohydrate, 5 mg cholesterol, 366 mg sodium.

saltsense: Omitting the salt reduces the sodium to 188 mg per serving.

curried navy beans

makes 8 servings

These curried beans, a hearty addition to any meal, go especially well with fish. Beans are almost miraculous. They're loaded with fiber, low in fat and can even help lower cholesterol levels. What more can you ask from a food? How about that it will also be easy to prepare? Just open a couple of cans and you're close to creating a healthful, substantial side dish.

2   medium baking (russet) potatoes, peeled and cut into ½-inch-thick pieces

3   15-ounce cans navy beans, drained, *divided*

1   cup fat-free reduced-sodium chicken broth (preferably homemade)

4   teaspoons peeled, minced fresh ginger

½   teaspoon turmeric

1   tablespoon olive oil

2   cups chopped onions

2   teaspoons hot curry powder, or to taste

1   cup chopped fresh tomato
    Salt and fresh-ground black pepper

½   cup chopped fresh cilantro

1.   Fill a medium saucepan two-thirds full of water and bring to a boil. Add the potatoes, reduce the heat to low and simmer until tender, about 15 minutes. Drain and set aside.

2.   In a food processor or blender, blend 1 cup of the beans with the broth, ginger and turmeric until smooth.

3.   Place a large nonstick skillet over medium-high heat and add the oil. When it is hot, sauté the onions until soft, about 5 minutes. Add the curry powder and cook, stirring, until fragrant, about 1 minute. Add the remaining 3 cups beans, the pureed beans,

 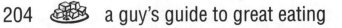

potatoes and tomato to the skillet. Reduce the heat to low and cook, stirring occasionally, until thick and creamy, about 5 minutes. Season with salt and pepper to taste. Transfer to a serving bowl and garnish with the cilantro. Serve immediately.

Nutritional information per serving (without added salt): 212 calories (10.5% from fat), 2.5 g fat (0.3 g saturated fat), 11.5 g protein, 37.5 g carbohydrate, 0 mg cholesterol, 314 mg sodium.

leansuggestion: Serve with Never-Better Roasted Pork Loin (page 86).

fancy sweet corn bread

makes 6 servings

This may be the best corn bread I've ever tasted. The buttermilk is essential, adding a sweet, tangy note that sets this quick bread apart.

1½ cups yellow cornmeal, preferably stoneground
½ cup unbleached all-purpose flour
3 tablespoons granulated sugar
2 teaspoons baking powder

½ teaspoon baking soda
1 large egg yolk
2 teaspoons canola oil
2 large egg whites
1½ cups low-fat buttermilk

1. Place the oven rack in the center, place an 8-by-8-by-2-inch baking pan on the rack and preheat the oven to 425 degrees.

2. In a medium mixing bowl, stir together the cornmeal, flour, sugar, baking powder and baking soda. Set aside.

3. In a large mixing bowl, whisk together the egg yolk and oil until combined. Add the egg whites and buttermilk and whisk until combined. Add the cornmeal mixture and stir until just moistened; the batter will not be smooth.

4. Carefully remove the preheated pan from the oven and place it on a heatproof surface. Lightly spray the pan with vegetable oil. Immediately pour the batter into the pan, smooth the top and bake for 25 minutes, or until the top is light brown and a toothpick inserted in the center comes out clean. Cool slightly and serve.

Nutritional information per serving: 229 calories (17.7% from fat), 4.5 g fat (0.6 g saturated fat), 6.7 g protein, 40.3 g carbohydrate, 36 mg cholesterol, 283 mg sodium.

 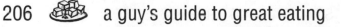

leansuggestions: When whisking in the buttermilk, you can add one of the following to the batter: ½ cup fresh or frozen whole kernel yellow corn, or ½ cup grated reduced-fat sharp cheddar cheese, or ¼ cup chopped onion and ¼ cup chopped green bell pepper or 1 chopped jalapeño.

- For a Carolina flavor boost, substitute 2 teaspoons bacon grease for the 2 teaspoons canola oil.
- Plain corn bread may be served with apple butter or strawberry preserves.

 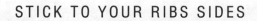

great green things

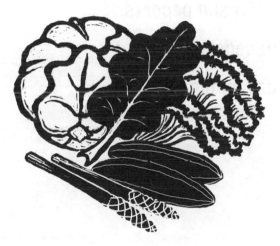

spicy oven-fried onion rings

steakhouse spinach

asparagus with parmesan cheese

east asian garlic broccoli

zucchini and carrots with garlic and basil

cabbage with corn and peppers

summertime vegetable ragout

sweet, sweet corn on the cob

There's a terrific steakhouse near

downtown Chicago called Gene and Georgetti's, where perfectly prepared prime beef is the specialty. Sautéed spinach is one of the few vegetables the restaurant offers. Bright green, toothsome and flavored with butter and garlic, it literally melts in your mouth. I duplicated this dish at home with much less fat and all the flavor. The result is a dish that Gene and Georgetti's would be proud to serve.

For most vegetables, simple is best. They should be impeccably fresh and in tip-top condition to start with. If they aren't, even elaborate preparations won't save them. If you've ever pulled a carrot out of the ground, rinsed it off and taken a bite, you know what I mean. A truly fresh carrot can be so sweet that it tastes sugary, unlike the woody orange sticks in a plastic bag at the supermarket.

This chapter wouldn't be complete without Spicy Oven-Fried Onion Rings, which I couldn't resist including even though they're not green. Most home cooks never make onion rings, preferring to leave them to restaurants, where deep fryers make them crisp—and full of grease.

I marinate my onion rings overnight in tangy low-fat buttermilk, then dip them in spicy toasted bread crumbs and bake them until they're golden brown and crunchy. They have a savory exterior and a sweet, soft interior. Best of all, oven-frying leaves no grease on your fingers, only a terrific taste in your mouth.

spicy oven-fried onion rings

makes about 20 onion rings

Once, when I was dining at a restaurant, some chili-seasoned fried onion rings were served as a garnish to my main dish. I was impressed with the contrast of spicy heat and sweet onion, and I vowed to recreate the dish at home, without all the grease of deep-frying. After innumerable tests, success: tons of flavor and practically zero fat.

3 cups fat-free or low-fat buttermilk
1 large sweet onion, such as a Vidalia or Texas Sweet, peeled, cut into ¼-inch-thick slices and separated into rings
2 cups dry unseasoned bread crumbs
2 teaspoons kosher salt
2 teaspoons paprika

1 teaspoon fresh-ground black pepper
1 teaspoon ground white pepper
1 teaspoon cayenne pepper
1 teaspoon chili powder

1. Place the buttermilk and onion rings in a 1-gallon recloseable plastic bag. Press out as much air as possible, seal and refrigerate for 3 hours or overnight.

2. Place the oven rack in the upper-middle position and preheat the oven to 400 degrees. Lightly spray a jelly-roll pan with vegetable oil and set aside.

3. Stir together the remaining ingredients in a medium mixing bowl.

4. Remove the onion rings, one at a time, from the bag and coat with the bread-crumb

mixture. Lay each ring on the prepared pan, making sure they do not touch. Lightly spray the rings with butter-flavored vegetable oil. Bake for 20 to 25 minutes, or until brown and crispy. Serve immediately.

Nutritional information per onion ring: 18 calories (18.4% from fat), 0.4 g fat (trace of saturated fat), 0.5 g protein, 2.2 g carbohydrate, trace of cholesterol, 37 mg sodium.

steakhouse spinach

makes 4 servings

At Gene and Georgetti's, a steakhouse near downtown Chicago, the sautéed spinach is as much of a draw as the fabulous steaks. Is my lean version as good as theirs? It's damn close.

1 tablespoon olive oil

2 medium garlic cloves, minced

2 pounds spinach leaves, stems removed, washed and spun in a salad spinner until very dry

Salt and fresh-ground black pepper

Place a 5-quart nonstick saucepan over medium-high heat and add the oil. When it is hot, add the garlic and sauté for 1 minute, or until softened. Add one-fourth of the spinach leaves to the saucepan, tossing with tongs. As the spinach wilts, add more spinach, tossing with the tongs, until it has all been added. Cook, tossing, until the spinach is completely wilted but still bright green, about 2 minutes. Remove from the heat and season to taste with salt and pepper. Serve immediately, using the tongs to squeeze out some of the moisture.

Nutritional information per serving (unsalted): 63 calories (53.5% from fat), 3.8 g fat (0.5 g saturated fat), 4.1 g protein, 5.7 g carbohydrate, 0 mg cholesterol, 106 mg sodium.

leansuggestion: Just a few drops of good balsamic vinegar on each serving add a terrific flavor to the spinach.

asparagus with parmesan cheese

makes 4 servings

When I lived in Illinois, I could barely wait until the Michigan asparagus hit my local farmer's market. This is my all-time favorite way to cook this great springtime vegetable. If possible, use imported Parmigiano-Reggiano cheese. It costs a little more but adds the perfect note to this simple yet sublime dish.

1 pound fresh asparagus, washed and trimmed

2 teaspoons Butter Buds, mixed with 2 tablespoons hot water

Fresh-ground black pepper to taste

2 tablespoons fresh-grated Parmesan cheese

1. Place the asparagus in a 12-inch skillet and add just enough water to cover. Cover and bring to a boil over high heat. When the water boils, remove from the heat immediately. Let stand for 1 minute. Drain.

2. Divide the asparagus among 4 dinner plates. Drizzle the Butter Buds liquid over each serving. Sprinkle Parmesan cheese over each serving and add pepper to taste. Serve immediately.

Nutritional information per serving: 40 calories (20.6% from fat), 0.9 g fat (0.5 g saturated fat), 4.5 g protein, 6.3 g carbohydrate, 2 mg cholesterol, 83.2 mg sodium.

cookingtip: After washing the asparagus, hold the top of each spear 2 inches below the tip and begin to bend from the bottom. The asparagus will snap and break at the point where it is tender. Discard the ends, which are tough.

east asian garlic broccoli

makes 4 servings

Soy sauce and garlic play up the flavor of broccoli perfectly. Don't be put off by the oyster sauce in this recipe. You've probably enjoyed it in Chinese restaurants for years. It's in most supermarkets in the Asian food section.

1½ pounds fresh broccoli
½   cup fat-free reduced-sodium
     chicken broth
3½ tablespoons oyster sauce
1½ tablespoons Scotch whisky
1   teaspoon reduced-sodium soy sauce
1¼ teaspoons toasted sesame oil, *divided*

2   teaspoons cornstarch
1   tablespoon peeled, grated fresh
     ginger
2   large garlic cloves, minced

1. Trim and discard the ends of the broccoli stems and cut the stems off just beneath the florets. Peel the tough outer skin from the stems and cut them, on the diagonal, into 1½-inch sections. Separate the florets into 1½-inch pieces. Set aside.

2. Whisk the broth, oyster sauce, whisky, soy sauce, ¼ teaspoon of the sesame oil and cornstarch in a small mixing bowl. Set aside.

3. Add 3 quarts water to a 5-quart pot and bring to a boil over high heat. Add the broccoli and return to a boil. Reduce the heat to low and simmer for 3 minutes, or until the broccoli is crisp-tender. Immediately drain in a colander and rinse under cold running water; drain thoroughly.

4. Heat a 12-inch cast-iron skillet over medium heat, and add the remaining 1 teaspoon sesame oil. When it is hot, add the ginger and garlic and sauté for 15 seconds, or until fragrant. Add the sauce to the skillet and cook, stirring constantly, until thickened, about 30 seconds. Add the broccoli, toss lightly to coat with the sauce and serve.

Nutritional information per serving: 86 calories (22.8% from fat), 2.2 g fat (0.2 g saturated fat), 4.2 g protein, 11.1 g carbohydrate, 0 mg cholesterol, 181 mg sodium.

leansuggestion: For a vegetarian meal, toss the broccoli and sauce with cooked linguine (from ¾ pound dried). I also like to add ¼ teaspoon Tabasco sauce or other hot sauce to the broccoli before tossing with the linguine. Oyster sauce is available in a vegetarian version.

 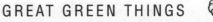 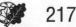

zucchini and carrots with garlic and basil

makes 4 servings

This dish is best in the middle of summer, when all the ingredients are fresh in local markets. A little muscle is necessary to squeeze out the water from the grated zucchini and carrots, making the result nice and crispy instead of soggy.

3 medium zucchini (about 1 pound total), trimmed and coarsely grated

2 medium carrots, peeled and coarsely grated

1 tablespoon olive oil

2 garlic cloves, minced

2 tablespoons minced fresh basil leaves

½ teaspoon salt, or to taste

¼ teaspoon fresh-ground black pepper

1. Layer 2 paper towels on the counter. Add half the shredded zucchini and carrots to the center of the towels. Bring together the four corners of the towels and lightly twist. Over the sink, squeeze the zucchini mixture hard several times (a tablespoon or so of liquid should drip out). Transfer the mixture to a bowl. Using fresh paper towels, squeeze the water out of the remaining zucchini mixture and add to the bowl.

2. Place a 10-inch nonstick skillet over medium-high heat and add the oil. When it is hot, add the zucchini mixture and garlic and cook, stirring occasionally, until tender, 4 to 6 minutes. Stir in the basil, salt and pepper. Serve immediately.

Nutritional information per serving: 60 calories (53% from fat), 3.5 g fat (0.5 g saturated fat), 1.3 g protein, 6.9 g carbohydrate, 0 mg cholesterol, 281 mg sodium.

 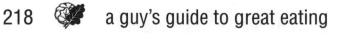

cabbage with corn and peppers

makes 6 servings

If it isn't overcooked, cabbage is pale green and sweet, and it doesn't make the whole house stink. I love cooking cabbage with onion, garlic, bell peppers, tomatoes and corn from my local farmer's market for a satisfying side dish. Use fresh dill if it is available, since it tastes better than dried.

- 2 teaspoons olive oil
- 2 garlic cloves, finely chopped
- 3 cups shredded green cabbage
- 2 medium tomatoes, peeled and cut into cubes
- 1 medium onion, thinly sliced
- 1 cup thinly sliced celery
- 1 cup corn kernels
- ½ cup chopped green bell pepper
- 1 tablespoon fresh dill leaves (or 1 teaspoon dried, crumbled)
- 1 teaspoon granulated sugar
- 1 teaspoon salt
- ½ teaspoon fresh-ground black pepper

Place a large nonstick skillet over medium heat and add the oil. When it is hot, add the garlic and cook for 1 minute, or until fragrant. Stir in the cabbage, tomatoes, onion, celery, corn, bell pepper, dill, sugar, salt and pepper. Cover and cook, stirring occasionally, for 6 to 8 minutes, until the cabbage wilts. Serve.

Nutritional information per serving: 75 calories (24.3% from fat), 2 g fat (0.3 g saturated fat), 2.5 g protein, 13.6 g carbohydrate, 0 mg cholesterol, 393 mg sodium.

saltsense: Reducing the salt to ½ teaspoon cuts back the sodium to 215 mg per serving.

summertime vegetable ragout

makes 4 servings

When I grill burgers or chicken breasts, I serve this exceptional vegetable ragout on the side. Fresh basil and oregano elevate the flavors.

1 tablespoon olive oil
1 medium onion, finely chopped
3 garlic cloves, minced
2 medium zucchini, ends trimmed, cut into ½-inch dice
1 medium yellow summer squash, ends trimmed, cut into ½-inch dice
1 red bell pepper, chopped
1 cup fresh corn kernels (cut from 1 large ear)

2 large ripe tomatoes, cut into ½-inch dice
2 tablespoons minced fresh oregano (or ½ teaspoon dried, crumbled)
½ teaspoon salt
½ teaspoon fresh-ground black pepper
½ cup packed fresh basil leaves, shredded

1. Place the oil in a large nonstick skillet over medium-low heat. When it is hot, add the onion and garlic and cook, stirring, until softened, about 5 minutes. Increase the heat to medium, add the zucchini, summer squash, bell pepper and corn and cook, stirring, for 4 minutes.

2. Add the tomatoes, oregano, salt and pepper, reduce the heat to low and simmer, covered, stirring occasionally, for 10 minutes. Uncover and simmer, stirring occasionally, for 5 minutes more, or until some of the moisture has evaporated. Sprinkle with the basil and serve warm or at room temperature.

Nutritional information per serving: 133 calories (29.2% from fat), 4.3 g fat (0.6 g saturated fat), 4 g protein, 22.7 g carbohydrate, 0 mg cholesterol, 286 mg sodium.

sweet, sweet corn on the cob

makes 6 servings

Sure, I've heard the story, too. If you want the sweetest corn on the planet, have the water boiling before going to the garden to pick the corn. Well, that's just dandy for folks who grow corn.

I've got a better way to ensure sweet corn on the cob. I buy the "supersweet" variety. (It's bred not to convert its natural sugar to carbohydrate quickly.) If I can't find supersweet, I cook the corn in honey-sweetened water. Then I serve it with a squeezable, fat-free margarine or lime wedges.

6 ears fresh sweet corn, shucked, silk removed and ends trimmed

⅓ cup clover or other mild honey (optional)

2 limes, quartered

1. Fill a large pot with enough water to cover the corn by at least 2 inches. Bring to a boil over high heat and whisk in the honey, if using.

2. Add the corn. When the water returns to a boil, remove from the heat, cover and let stand for 4 to 5 minutes, or until the corn is tender. (Older ears will take longer, 7 to 9 minutes. Extremely fresh corn will be done in about 4 minutes.)

3. Using long-handled tongs, remove the corn, allowing the water to drip off, and serve immediately with the lime wedges on the side.

Nutritional information per (unsalted) ear: 83 calories (10.8% from fat), 1 g fat (0.2 g saturated fat), 2.6 g protein, 19.3 g carbohydrate, 0 mg cholesterol, 13 mg sodium.

slaws
n' salads

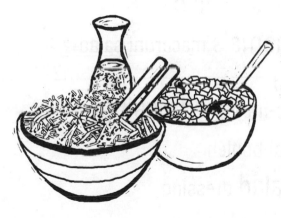

carolina slaw

sour cream cabbage slaw

summer slaw

real american creamy potato salad

"delish" potato salad

summertime potato salad

not-your-mama's macaroni salad

one-bean salad
        with lime-mustard dressing

couscous tabbouleh

caesar-style salad dressing

slightly thickened chicken broth

ranch-style salad dressing

real bacon salad dressing

roasted garlic salad dressing

If I've heard it once, I've heard it a hundred times: men like meat, women like salads. Well, that might be the case if you're talking about some frilly little fruit salad, but it's certainly not true of one of my potato salads or cabbage slaws.

My Carolina Slaw is every bit as good as the ones served at barbecue joints throughout the Carolinas. The dressing for Sour Cream Cabbage Slaw is zinged with horseradish and has zero mayonnaise and very little fat. In Summer Slaw, low-fat mayonnaise, clover honey and two kinds of wine vinegar unite in a perfectly balanced dressing for the vegetables that abound at farm stands in the summer.

Each of the potato salads in this chapter meets or exceeds my stringent reduced-fat standards. Real American Creamy Potato Salad is worthy of being piled on a summer picnic plate next to some cold oven-fried chicken and sliced homegrown tomatoes. "Delish" Potato Salad, another irresistible creamy version, is based on a recipe from an unusually good Chicago deli, while Summertime Potato Salad includes all the good things of that season: new potatoes, cherry tomatoes, red onions, corn and fresh basil.

For all slaws and salads, the dressing makes the difference, since almost all of the fat and calories lurk here. I didn't gain all that weight by eating vegetables, and to keep it off, I've learned to make my own dressings from low-fat mayonnaise (1 fat gram per tablespoon versus 11 in the full-fat kind), reduced-fat sour cream (3.5 fat grams per 2 tablespoons versus 5 grams for regular) or flavorful, slightly thickened chicken broth, which I substitute for most of the oil.

The flavors of these salads depend on excellent ingredients, not fat. Whether you serve them with lunch or dinner, on the picnic table or at the dinner table, you can be sure that the staunchest meat lover will make room on his plate.

carolina slaw

makes 8 servings

North Carolina slaw is made with mayonnaise—no surprise—but also with vinegar. This slaw goes well with any summer meal, from burgers to chicken, and makes the perfect topping for a North Carolina Pulled Turkey Barbecue (page 116) sandwich.

1 cup low-fat mayonnaise (1 fat gram per tablespoon)

2 tablespoons cider vinegar

1 tablespoon clover or other mild honey

1 teaspoon celery seeds

½ teaspoon salt, or to taste

¼ teaspoon fresh-ground black pepper

1 head (about 1½ pounds) green cabbage, finely shredded

3 scallions, white and green parts, chopped

1 carrot, peeled and coarsely grated

In a large mixing bowl, whisk together the mayonnaise, vinegar, honey, celery seeds, salt and pepper. Add the cabbage, scallions and carrot and stir until coated with the dressing. Cover and chill before serving.

Nutritional information per serving: 86 calories (26.8% from fat), 2.6 g fat (trace of saturated fat), 2.5 g protein, 16.1 g carbohydrate, 0 mg cholesterol, 439 mg sodium.

cookingtip: To keep the slaw crisp when making it in advance: Sprinkle the cabbage and carrot with 2 teaspoons kosher salt or 1 teaspoon regular salt and toss. Place in a colander and put the colander in the sink. Set aside for 1 hour or up to 4 hours, or until the cabbage wilts. Rinse under cold water and spin-dry in batches in a salad spinner. Proceed as directed.

saltsense: Omitting the salt reduces the sodium to 305 mg per serving.

sour cream cabbage slaw

makes 8 servings

This slaw was inspired by a recipe from James Beard, who said he got it from someone in Minnesota. The horseradish was his — and my — favorite addition. Of course, Beard used full-fat sour cream for his version. (He didn't get that big by eating light.) My leaner version tastes just as delicious as Beard's.

½ cup reduced-fat sour cream
½ cup nonfat sour cream
3 tablespoons cider vinegar
1½ tablespoons clover or other mild honey
1 tablespoon chopped fresh dill, or more to taste
2 teaspoons prepared horseradish

1 teaspoon salt
1 teaspoon fresh-ground black pepper
1 teaspoon dry mustard (preferably Colman's)
1 2-pound green cabbage, shredded or chopped

1. In a small bowl, whisk together all the ingredients except the cabbage. Cover and chill for 1 to 2 hours to let the flavors blend and mellow.

2. Place the cabbage in a large mixing bowl, add the dressing and stir until the cabbage is coated. Cover and chill for 1 hour before serving.

Nutritional information per serving: 85 calories (23.5% from fat), 2.2 g fat (1.3 g saturated fat), 4.9 g protein, 13.8 g carbohydrate, 9.6 mg cholesterol, 321 mg sodium.

cookingtips: The dressing and cabbage may be mixed together, covered and chilled for 1 to 2 hours before serving. Toss just before serving.

- You can substitute 3 packets of artificial sweetener (equal to 2 tablespoons granulated sugar) for the honey.

summer slaw

makes 12 servings

In midsummer, when cabbage makes its appearance at farmer's markets, along with bell peppers, fresh dill and carrots, it's time to make one of my favorite slaws. The dressing is a creamy oil-and-vinegar version, minus most of the fat of the original.

dressing

- 1¾ cups low-fat mayonnaise (1 fat gram per tablespoon)
- 3 tablespoons clover or other mild honey
- 1 tablespoon red wine vinegar
- 1 tablespoon white wine vinegar
- ½ teaspoon fresh-ground black pepper
- ¼ teaspoon celery seeds
- ¼ teaspoon fresh garlic, minced

salad

- 1 large (about 4 pounds) green cabbage, shredded
- ½ cup coarsely grated carrot
- ½ cup fine-chopped green bell pepper
- ½ cup fine-chopped red bell pepper
- ½ cup fine-chopped celery
- 3 tablespoons fine-chopped red onion
- 1½ teaspoons fine-chopped fresh dill
- 1½ teaspoons fine-chopped fresh parsley leaves

1. **To make the dressing:** In a large bowl, whisk together all the ingredients.
2. **To assemble the salad:** Add the vegetables and herbs to the bowl. Stir until evenly coated with the dressing. Cover and chill for at least 4 hours or overnight before serving.

Nutritional information per serving: 119 calories (23.5% from fat), 3.1 g fat (trace of saturated fat), 4.3 g protein, 23 g carbohydrate, 0 mg cholesterol, 369 mg sodium.

leansuggestion: Just before serving, add ¾ cup peeled, seeded, diced fresh plum tomatoes and toss to combine.

cookingtip: If you plan to make the salad in advance, see the tip on page 226.

 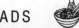

real american creamy potato salad

makes 12 servings.

Sweet onions appear from Vidalia, Georgia, in early summer. Most supermarkets carry Vidalias when they are in season, and they bring a sweet-sharp dimension to this salad. Yellow mustard is the classic, but if you prefer Dijon or some other mustard, use it instead. When I think of warm summer breezes and a picnic table loaded with great summer foods, this potato salad comes to mind.

3 pounds medium red-skin potatoes, scrubbed

1½ cups low-fat mayonnaise (1 fat gram per tablespoon)

2 tablespoons chopped fresh parsley

1½ teaspoons prepared yellow mustard

1 teaspoon salt

½ teaspoon fresh-ground black pepper

1 medium sweet onion, such as Vidalia or Texas Sweet, finely chopped

4 celery ribs, strings removed and diced

1. Bring a large pot of water to a boil, add the potatoes and cook for 25 minutes, or until they can be easily pierced with a knife but the interior offers a bit of resistance. Drain, cool and refrigerate. When the potatoes are chilled, cut them into ¼-inch cubes, leaving the skins on.

2. In a large bowl, whisk together the mayonnaise, parsley, mustard, salt and pepper. Add the potatoes, onion and celery and stir until coated with the dressing. Cover and chill for 2 hours before serving.

 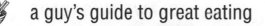

Nutritional information per serving: 182 calories (12.2% from fat), 2.5 g fat (trace of saturated fat), 2.9 g protein, 38.4 g carbohydrate, 0 mg cholesterol, 506 mg sodium.

leansuggestion: Mix the chopped whites of 3 hard-boiled eggs into the salad for egg flavor without fat.

saltsense: Omitting the salt reduces the sodium per serving to 324 mg.

"delish" potato salad

makes 12 servings

Many years ago in Chicago, there was a sensational deli named Delish within a few blocks of my office that prepared a potato salad I found irresistible. After the *Chicago Sun-Times* published the recipe, I recreated it. The original had almost 20 grams of fat per serving; my version has less than 3.

4 pounds new potatoes, scrubbed, each cut into ¼-inch-thick slices

1½ cups low-fat mayonnaise (1 fat gram per tablespoon)

1 cup diced celery

1 small bunch scallions, white parts only, thinly sliced

1 tablespoon paprika

1 tablespoon celery seeds

½ teaspoon salt

¼ teaspoon fresh-ground black pepper

6 large hard-cooked eggs, yolks discarded, whites coarsely chopped

1. Bring 2 inches of water to a boil in a large pot with a steamer basket in place. Place the potato slices in the basket and steam for 20 minutes, or until tender. Cool, cover and refrigerate for 1 to 2 hours, or until thoroughly chilled.

2. In a large bowl, whisk together the mayonnaise, celery, scallions, paprika, celery seeds, salt and pepper. Add the potatoes and egg whites and toss gently to coat. Cover and chill for 2 hours before serving.

 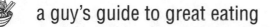

Nutritional information per serving: 197 calories (12.2% from fat), 2.7 g fat (trace of saturated fat), 4.1 g protein, 39.6 g carbohydrate, 0 mg cholesterol, 423 mg sodium.

cooking**tips**: Instead of steaming the sliced potatoes, you can boil them in water to cover for 15 minutes, or until a knife pierces them easily. Drain, chill and slice into ¼-inch-thick rounds. Proceed as directed.

- ◆   This salad tastes best when served within 24 hours of preparation.

leansuggestion: For a Chicago-style Swedish variation, substitute 1 tablespoon of caraway seeds for the celery seeds.

summertime potato salad

makes 8 servings

Three vegetables scream summer: tomatoes, corn and small new red potatoes. This salad is best eaten the day it is prepared, since it gets watery if it sits too long.

3 pounds small, new red-skin potatoes, scrubbed
1¼ cup nonfat mayonnaise
⅓ cup unseasoned rice vinegar (or white wine vinegar)
1 tablespoon granulated sugar
½ teaspoon salt
¼ teaspoon fresh-ground black pepper

1½ pounds ripe plum tomatoes, peeled, seeded and cut into ¾-inch pieces
1 cup cooked corn kernels (from 1 ear of corn)
1 cup chopped red onion
1 cup chopped fresh basil leaves

1. Bring a large pot of water to a boil, add the potatoes and cook until they can be easily pierced with a knife, about 20 minutes. Drain. Set aside until cool enough to handle. Cut the potatoes into ¼-inch-thick slices.

2. In a large bowl, whisk together the mayonnaise, vinegar, sugar, salt and pepper. Add the potatoes, tomatoes, corn, onion and basil, stirring until coated with the dressing. Cover and chill for 2 hours before serving.

a guy's guide to great eating

Nutritional information per serving: 235 calories (2.8% from fat), 0.7 g fat (trace of saturated fat), 3.8 g protein, 55 g carbohydrate, 0 mg cholesterol, 638 mg sodium.

cooking**tip**: Rice vinegar is available at supermarkets with the other vinegars or in the Chinese food section.

saltsense: Omitting the salt reduces the sodium to 505 mg per serving.

not-your-mama's macaroni salad

makes 8 servings

One day, I was fooling around with some elbow macaroni and created this salad. People tell me it's the one they remember from childhood. This salad keeps well.

1½ teaspoons salt
½ pound dried elbow macaroni
1 cup low-fat mayonnaise (1 fat gram per tablespoon)
¼ cup nonfat sour cream
1½ teaspoons celery seeds
½ teaspoon fresh-ground black pepper
2 tablespoons sweet pickle juice (from the pickle jar)
1 large tomato, peeled, seeded and coarsely chopped

4 sweet or bread-and-butter pickles, coarsely chopped
½ red bell pepper, finely chopped
1 bunch scallions, white and green parts, finely chopped
¼ cup chopped fresh parsley leaves
2 tablespoons fresh dill (or 2 teaspoons dried, crumbled)

1. Bring 5 quarts water to a rolling boil in a large pot. Stir in the salt. Add the macaroni and stir until the water returns to a boil. Reduce the heat slightly and boil for 8 to 10 minutes, or until a noodle offers a little resistance when bitten. Drain and rinse with cold water. Set aside.

2. In a medium bowl, whisk together the mayonnaise, sour cream, celery seeds, pepper and pickle juice.

3. Add the remaining ingredients and the macaroni to the bowl. Stir until evenly coated with the dressing. Cover and refrigerate for 2 hours before serving.

Nutritional information per serving: 197 calories (17.3% from fat), 3.8 g fat (0.7 g saturated fat), 4.1 g protein, 36.9 g carbohydrate, 4 mg cholesterol, 437 mg sodium.

one-bean salad with lime-mustard dressing

makes 6 servings

My wife created this lime-mustard dressing, based on one she saw in a seed catalog. It's a great match for fresh green beans.

1 pound fresh green beans, ends trimmed
2 tablespoons coarse Dijon mustard
2 tablespoons rice vinegar or white wine vinegar
  Juice of 1 lime
1 tablespoon olive oil
½ teaspoon clover or other mild honey (or use a sugar substitute equivalent to ½ teaspoon sugar)

1 garlic clove, minced
1 large shallot, minced
½ teaspoon minced lime peel
  Salt and fresh-ground black pepper to taste

1. Fill a 5-to-6-quart saucepan half full with water and bring to a rolling boil. Add the green beans and stir until the water returns to a boil. Cook, uncovered, for 3 to 4 minutes, or until the beans become bright green and crisp-tender. Drain and immediately plunge the beans into ice water to stop the cooking; drain well.

2. In a medium bowl, whisk together the remaining ingredients, adding salt and pepper to taste.

3. Add the beans to the dressing, and toss to coat. Let stand for 30 minutes, tossing occasionally, then serve.

Nutritional information per serving (without added salt): 54 calories (44.8% from fat), 2.6 g fat (0.3 g saturated fat), 1 g protein, 6.8 g carbohydrate, 0 mg cholesterol, 116 mg sodium.

couscous tabbouleh

makes 6 servings

Tabbouleh, the Middle Eastern salad, tastes great, but finding bulgur wheat, its traditional foundation, can be a problem. I decided to make it with couscous, which is a cinch to find. (It's located near the rice in supermarkets.) Fresh mint makes all the flavors sparkle.

1 cup fat-free reduced-sodium chicken broth
¾ cup couscous
1 cup chopped fresh flat-leaf parsley
2 large tomatoes, finely chopped
1 red onion, finely chopped
3 tablespoons chopped fresh mint leaves
3 tablespoons Slightly Thickened Chicken Broth (page 240)

3 tablespoons fresh-squeezed lemon juice, or to taste
3 garlic cloves, minced
1 tablespoon olive oil
½ teaspoon fresh-ground black pepper
½ teaspoon salt, or to taste

1. In a small saucepan, bring the broth to a boil over medium-high heat and stir in the couscous. Cover and remove from the heat. Let stand for 5 minutes. Transfer the couscous to a medium mixing bowl, fluff with a fork and let cool to room temperature.

2. Add the remaining ingredients to the couscous and toss to coat. Cover and refrigerate for 1 hour to allow the flavors to blend. Remove from the refrigerator 30 minutes before serving.

Nutritional information per serving: 143 calories (18% from fat), 2.9 g fat (0.4 g saturated fat), 5.3 g protein, 25.6 g carbohydrate, 0 mg cholesterol, 291 mg sodium.

caesar-style salad dressing

makes 2 cups

Despite the fact that all the ingredients of a classic Caesar salad are healthful, the dressing delivers a high-fat wallop. But what's a Caesar salad without the dressing? Just a bunch of romaine lettuce. The only thing missing from my lean version is 12 grams of fat per table-spoon. I take a bottle of my dressing along with me to my favorite restaurant. I order the Caesar salad, sans dressing, with a sliced broiled chicken breast on top. Then I take out my dressing and pour it on.

6 tablespoons red wine vinegar	1½ teaspoons Worcestershire sauce
¼ cup fat-free egg substitute	½ teaspoon Tabasco sauce
10 anchovy fillets, chopped and mashed	½ teaspoon fresh-ground black pepper
1 ounce fresh-grated Parmesan cheese	
1 tablespoon fresh-squeezed lemon juice	2 tablespoons extra-virgin olive oil
2 garlic cloves, mashed to a paste	1 cup Slightly Thickened Chicken
1½ teaspoons Dijon mustard	Broth (page 240)

Place the vinegar, egg substitute, anchovies, Parmesan cheese, lemon juice, garlic, mustard, Worcestershire sauce, Tabasco sauce and pepper in a medium mixing bowl and whisk until combined. Add the olive oil in a stream, whisking. Add the chicken broth in a stream, whisking. Cover and refrigerate for at least 1 hour before serving. The dressing will keep, refrigerated, for 7 to 10 days.

Nutritional information per 2 tablespoons: 34 calories (64% from fat), 2.4 g fat (0.6 g saturated fat), 1.8 g protein, 1 g carbohydrate, 3.6 mg cholesterol, 158 mg sodium.

slightly thickened chicken broth

makes about 1 cup

This recipe is an excellent substitute for oil in salad dressings. The difference? Only 63 calories instead of 1,900 and no fat whatsoever.

1 cup fat-free reduced-sodium chicken broth, *divided*

1 tablespoon plus 2 teaspoons cornstarch

Bring all but 2 tablespoons of broth to a boil in a small saucepan over high heat. Meanwhile, whisk together the 2 tablespoons broth and cornstarch. Gradually whisk the cornstarch mixture into the boiling broth. Boil until the broth is slightly thickened, about 30 seconds. Let cool before serving.

Nutritional information per tablespoon: 4 calories (0% from fat), trace of fat (trace of saturated fat), 0.1 g protein, 0.9 g carbohydrate, 0 mg cholesterol, 25 mg sodium.

cookingtip: Vegetable broth may be substituted for the chicken broth.

ranch-style salad dressing

makes 2½ cups

This dressing not only adds spark to a salad but also makes a super dip for fresh vegetables. It has about half the calories and just one-sixth of the fat of the traditional version.

¾ cup nonfat sour cream
¾ cup low-fat mayonnaise (1 fat gram per tablespoon)
½ cup low-fat buttermilk
2 tablespoons red wine vinegar
2¼ teaspoons Worcestershire sauce
2 teaspoons fresh-squeezed lemon juice

1½ teaspoons chopped fresh parsley
1½ teaspoons chopped fresh chives
1½ teaspoons minced shallot
1½ teaspoons Dijon mustard
1 garlic clove, mashed to a paste
½ teaspoon celery seeds
½ teaspoon salt

Whisk together all the ingredients and 2 tablespoons water in a small bowl. Refrigerate for at least 1 hour before serving. The dressing will keep, refrigerated, for 10 days.

Nutritional information per 2 tablespoons: 30 calories (22.9% from fat), 0.8 g fat (trace of saturated fat), 0.8 g protein, 4.6 g carbohydrate, 1.6 mg cholesterol, 140 mg sodium.

saltsense: Omitting the salt will reduce the sodium to 87 mg.

real bacon salad dressing

makes 1¾ cups

Adding oven-roasted bacon to a creamy, lean, French-style salad dressing gives you the best of both worlds: few calories, big flavor. Try it drizzled over a bowl of chopped iceberg lettuce.

1½ teaspoons dry mustard (preferably Colman's)
¼ cup fat-free reduced-sodium chicken broth, *divided*
¾ cup low-fat mayonnaise (1 fat gram per tablespoon)
3 pieces Oven-Roasted Bacon (page 12) trimmed of all visible fat and finely chopped

¼ cup red wine vinegar
1 tablespoon clover or other mild honey (or 2 packets sugar substitute)
1 tablespoon paprika
1 small garlic clove, minced

Place the mustard and 1 tablespoon of the broth in a medium mixing bowl and stir until it forms a paste. Whisk in the remaining broth and the rest of the ingredients. Taste and adjust the seasonings. Cover and refrigerate for 1 hour before serving. The dressing will keep, refrigerated, for 10 days.

Nutritional information per 2 tablespoons: 33 calories (34% from fat), 1.3 g fat (trace of saturated fat), 0.6 g protein, 5.4 g carbohydrate, trace of cholesterol, 151 mg sodium.

leansuggestion: Topping this salad with slices of grilled, skinless, boneless chicken breast makes it a meal.

roasted garlic salad dressing

makes about 2¼ cups

When I feel indulgent, I throw a lean flank steak on the grill and whisk together this lean version of the roasted garlic dressing often served in steakhouses.

1½ cups low-fat mayonnaise (1 fat gram per tablespoon)

½ cup nonfat sour cream

1 tablespoon plus 1 teaspoon Easy Sweet Oven-Roasted Garlic (page 192)

1 tablespoon chopped fresh oregano (or 1 teaspoon dried, crumbled)

1¼ teaspoons Dijon mustard

¼ teaspoon Tabasco sauce

¼ teaspoon fresh-ground black pepper

In a medium bowl, whisk together all the ingredients and ¼ cup water. Cover and refrigerate for 1 hour before serving. This dressing will keep, refrigerated, for 1 week.

Nutritional information per 2 tablespoons: 44 calories (32% from fat), 1.5 g fat (trace of saturated fat), 0.4 g protein, 7 g carbohydrate, 0.8 mg cholesterol, 209 mg sodium.

cooking**tip**: If this dressing is too thick, thin it with water.

the
munchies

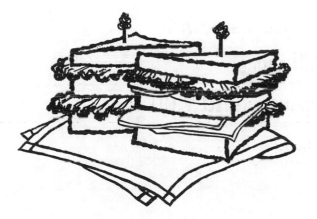

salsa mediterranean

sassy salsa with horseradish

black, white and red salsa

peanut butter hummus

bagels with sun-dried-tomato
cream cheese and salmon

carolina don's sub sandwich

hot dog chili sauce

classic clubhouse sandwich

pizza in a flash

You know the feeling:

you're ravenous and dinner won't be ready for an hour. Anyone can eat healthfully when there's plenty of time to cook. It's when you're starving that the chips are down. Take dips, for example. Most of them are loaded with fat and calories. To cut the fat drastically, I use low-fat mayonnaise or reduced-fat or nonfat sour cream and cream cheese in all my favorite dips.

Or I whip up my own salsa, which makes the bottled kind seem weak sister. Black, White and Red Salsa is a sassy blend of black and white beans, red bell peppers and red onions, corn, garlic and jalapeño peppers. But in place of the whopping ¾ cup of oil that I once used, I substitute full-flavored chicken broth, cutting almost 1,500 calories and 180 fat grams.

When I want something fast for lunch, the sandwich is king. But because in most lunch places the only way to save on fat grams is to remove some of the ingredients, I set up shop in my own kitchen and build my big sandwich exactly how I want it. I generously smear mustard and low-fat mayonnaise on French bread and layer on paper-thin slices of pepperoni, salami, ham, fat-free bologna and provolone cheese. Finally, I pile on the onions, lettuce, green peppers, jalapeños and tomato slices for a fast, low-fat feast.

Do these snacks sound ridiculously easy to you? That's just the point.

salsa mediterranean

makes 2 cups

One day I asked myself why there isn't a salsa that reflects the flavors of the Mediterranean. To make one, I added Dijon mustard and substituted basil for cilantro. Instead of tortilla chips, I toasted wedges of pita bread.

2 tablespoons Dijon mustard
2 tablespoons white wine vinegar
1½ teaspoons red wine vinegar
1 teaspoon olive oil
2 cups diced tomatoes
1 cup chopped fresh basil leaves

2 garlic cloves, minced
½ teaspoon salt
½ teaspoon fresh-ground black pepper

Toasted pita bread wedges

In a medium bowl, whisk together the mustard, vinegars and oil. Stir in the tomatoes, basil, garlic, salt and pepper. Serve with the toasted pita bread wedges.

Nutritional information per tablespoon: 5 calories (43.5% from fat), 0.2 g fat (trace of saturated fat), trace of protein, 0.6 g carbohydrate, 0 mg cholesterol, 62 mg sodium.

cookingtip: To make the pita bread wedges: Place the oven rack in the lower-middle position and preheat the oven to 375 degrees. Split 6 pita breads and cut each round into 6 or 8 wedges. Place on a jelly-roll pan, sprinkle with a little kosher salt and bake for 10 to 12 minutes, or until crisp. Serve immediately. Repeat with the remaining wedges. Makes 36 to 48 wedges.

 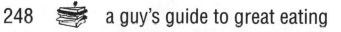

sassy salsa with horseradish

makes about 3 cups

This salsa uses sinus-clearing horseradish and Tabasco for moderate heat. Fresh plum tomatoes can be substituted for canned when they're in season.

- 1 28-ounce can plum tomatoes, drained and chopped
- 1 4-ounce can chopped mild green chilies
- ½ cup fine-chopped onion
- 1 large garlic clove, finely chopped
- 1 teaspoon drained bottled horseradish
- ¼ teaspoon fresh-ground black pepper
- ¼ teaspoon Tabasco sauce
- ½ teaspoon salt

Place all the ingredients, except the salt, in a medium mixing bowl and stir until combined. Cover and chill for 1 hour. Stir in the salt and adjust the seasonings just before serving.

Nutritional information per tablespoon: 5 calories (12.6% from fat), 0.07 g fat (trace of saturated fat), 0.2 g protein, 1 g carbohydrates, 0 mg cholesterol, 57 mg sodium.

cooking**tip**: Adding the salt just before serving prevents the salsa from getting watery.

leansuggestion: Serve this salsa on grilled beef or turkey burgers. It's also terrific on baked beans or other canned beans, and it makes a tasty topping for baked potatoes.

black, white and red salsa

makes about 6 cups

This salsa looks so beautiful that some folks hate to dip in. But once they do, they keep dipping until it's all gone.

1 15-ounce can black beans, rinsed and drained	2 tablespoons fresh-squeezed lime juice
1 15-ounce can Great Northern beans, rinsed and drained	1 tablespoon minced fresh oregano (or 1 teaspoon dried, crumbled)
1½ cups frozen corn kernels	1 tablespoon chili powder
1 cup chopped red bell pepper	3 garlic cloves, minced
¾ cup chopped red onion	1½ teaspoons ground cumin
¾ cup fat-free reduced-sodium chicken broth	1 teaspoon salt
1 large jalapeño pepper, seeded and minced	½ teaspoon fresh-ground black pepper

Place all the ingredients in a large mixing bowl and stir until combined. Cover and refrigerate for 1 hour to allow the flavors to blend. Stir well and serve.

Nutritional information per tablespoon: 12 calories (5% from fat), trace of fat (0 g saturated fat), 0.7 g protein, 2.4 g carbohydrate, 0 mg cholesterol, 50 mg sodium.

leansuggestion: This salsa makes a terrific fat-free filling for burritos. Use fat-free flour tortillas, and add some grated reduced-fat Monterey Jack cheese. Warm in a microwave oven.

peanut butter hummus

makes about 4 cups

A couple of years ago, I wanted to make a batch of hummus, the popular Middle Eastern dip, and discovered I was out of tahini. Off to the supermarket I went but couldn't find it anywhere, so I bought reduced-fat peanut butter instead. My hummus tasted just like the traditional version. Now you, too, can make great hummus at home without searching far and wide for the ingredients.

- 1 large garlic clove
- 2 15-ounce cans chickpeas (garbanzo beans), drained (reserve the liquid)
- ¼ cup plain nonfat yogurt
- 3 tablespoons fresh-squeezed lemon juice
- 2 tablespoons reduced-fat peanut butter

- 2 teaspoons olive oil
- 2 teaspoons toasted sesame seed oil
- 1 teaspoon ground cumin
- 1 teaspoon salt

With the motor running, drop the garlic clove through the feed tube of a food processor fitted with the steel blade. When it is finely chopped, stop the motor and add the chickpeas. Process for 30 seconds. With the processor running, add the yogurt, lemon juice, peanut butter, olive oil, sesame oil, cumin and salt. Process, stopping from time to time to scrape down the bowl, until smooth. If the hummus is too thick or dry, thin with some of the reserved chickpea liquid. Taste and adjust the seasonings. Serve.

Nutritional information per tablespoon: 17 calories (30.5% from fat), 0.6 g fat (0.08 g saturated fat), 1 g protein, 2.4 g carbohydrate, 0 mg cholesterol, 46 mg sodium.

bagels with sun-dried-tomato cream cheese and salmon

makes 6 servings

Bagels and lox disappeared from my food plan when I lost weight, until I tasted a low-fat sun-dried-tomato dip at a party that I longed to pair with lox. I substituted leftover cold broiled salmon, and now I make enough salmon for leftovers every time.

¼ cup sun-dried tomatoes (not packed in oil)

4 ounces Neufchâtel cheese, at room temperature

4 ounces fat-free cream cheese, at room temperature

3 tablespoons sliced scallions, white and light green parts

6 plain bagels

9 ounces cold broiled salmon fillet, skin removed

Fresh-ground black pepper

1. Bring 1 cup water to a boil in a small saucepan. Place the sun-dried tomatoes in a small bowl and cover with the boiling water. Soak for 15 minutes, or until soft.

2. Meanwhile, place the cheeses in a food processor with the steel blade in place and process, pulsing, for 15 seconds, or until smooth. Scrape down the bowl.

3. Drain the sun-dried tomatoes and pat dry with paper towels. Add the tomatoes to the food processor and process, pulsing, for 10 to 20 seconds, scraping down the bowl if necessary, until the tomatoes have been chopped into small pieces.

4. Transfer the mixture to a medium bowl and stir in the scallions. Cover and refrigerate for 30 minutes.

 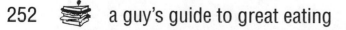

5.   Cut the bagels in half. Divide the cream cheese mixture among the bagels, spreading it evenly. Slice the salmon across the grain into thin slices. Place the salmon slices on the bagel bottoms, grind on pepper to taste and cover with the bagel tops. Serve immediately.

Nutritional information per sandwich: 366 calories (24% from fat), 9.7 g fat (3.3 g saturated fat), 24.3 g protein, 44.1 g carbohydrate, 46 mg cholesterol, 849 mg sodium.

saltsense: Using salt-free bagels will cut the sodium content by half.

 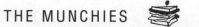

carolina don's sub sandwich

makes 1 serving

Paper-thin slices of meat are the key for me to be able to indulge in sub-style sandwiches. Since the sodium content of deli meats is high, cutting the fat also reduces the sodium.

1   tablespoon low-fat mayonnaise (1 fat gram per tablespoon)
1   6-inch length soft French bread, sliced in half horizontally
1   tablespoon prepared yellow mustard
2   slices fat-free bologna
2   paper-thin slices (0.8 ounce) baked ham
2   paper-thin slices (0.4 ounce) large-diameter pepperoni
2   paper-thin slices (0.3 ounce) Genoa salami

1   paper-thin slice (0.3 ounce) provolone cheese
4   thin green bell pepper rings
1   thin slice onion, separated into rings
8   thin slices jalapeño pepper
1   cup shredded lettuce
4   thin slices ripe tomato
    Salt and fresh-ground black pepper

Spread the mayonnaise on the top half of the bread. Spread the mustard on the bottom half. On the bottom half, layer the bologna, ham, pepperoni, salami, provolone, bell pepper, onion and jalapeño. Distribute the shredded lettuce over all, and top with the tomato slices. Sprinkle with salt and pepper to taste and serve.

Nutritional information per sub: 537 calories (26.1% from fat), 15.6 g fat (4.3 g saturated fat), 29.4 g protein, 66.7 g carbohydrate, 50 mg cholesterol, 2562 mg sodium.

hot dog chili sauce

makes enough sauce to top 6 hot dogs

I started making a chili sauce for hot dogs to bring back the taste of the past. It's equally excellent on a burger made of 93 percent lean meat.

1 teaspoon canola oil
½ cup chopped onion (preferably a sweet onion, such as Vidalia or Texas Sweet)
2 garlic cloves, minced
¾ pound 93% lean ground beef
¼ cup tomato ketchup
¼ cup tomato juice
1 tablespoon prepared yellow mustard

1 tablespoon white vinegar
1 teaspoon Worcestershire sauce
½ teaspoon Tabasco sauce, or to taste
½ teaspoon fresh-ground black pepper
¼ teaspoon salt

1. Place a large nonstick skillet over medium heat and add the oil. When it is hot, add the onion and garlic and cook, stirring, until softened, about 6 minutes.

2. Add the ground beef, breaking it up with the edge of a spoon, until cooked through, 6 to 7 minutes. (There should be no lumps; the meat should look like grains of rice in size and texture.) Drain off the fat.

3. Stir in the remaining ingredients, reduce the heat to low and simmer, stirring occasionally, for 10 minutes, or until slightly thickened.

Nutritional information per serving (with no salt added): 106 calories (32.9% from fat), 3.8 g fat (1.2 g saturated fat), 12.3 g protein, 5.5 g carbohydrate, 31 mg cholesterol, 323 mg sodium.

classic clubhouse sandwich

makes 1 sandwich

The classic club sandwich has lots of full-fat mayonnaise and is three layers high, with frilly toothpicks holding everything together. From a health perspective, there's a problem with the club, and it's not the toothpicks. The mayo alone brings along 44 fat grams and 400 calories. Add three or four slices of bacon, and the fat and calories zoom.

    I use low-fat mayonnaise and cut the fat grams to just 4. Oven-roasted bacon is far leaner than fried, and chicken breast is almost fat-free. Once you try this sandwich, you'll never go back to the other version.

4 tablespoons low-fat mayonnaise (1 fat gram per tablespoon), *divided*

3 slices good-quality white sandwich bread, lightly toasted

4 lettuce leaves, washed and dried, *divided*

2 thin slices tomato

4 slices Oven-Roasted Bacon (page 12), trimmed of all visible fat, at room temperature

½ cooked and chilled skinless, boneless chicken breast (page 95), sliced paper-thin across the grain

Salt and fresh-ground black pepper to taste

Sweet pickle chips

Baked potato crisps

1. Spread 1 tablespoon mayonnaise on each slice of bread. Lay a lettuce leaf on the first slice. Top the lettuce leaf with the tomato slices and another lettuce leaf. Place the second slice of bread, mayonnaise side down, on the lettuce leaf. Spread the last tablespoon of mayonnaise on the top side of the bread. Place a lettuce leaf on top, then the bacon and chicken. Sprinkle the chicken with the salt and pepper. Top with the remaining lettuce leaf. Place the remaining slice of bread on the lettuce leaf, mayonnaise side down.

 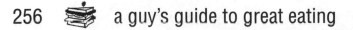

2. Pierce the sandwich with toothpicks ½ inch from each edge and cut it diagonally into quarters. Serve with the sweet pickle slices and baked potato crisps.

Nutritional information per sandwich (without added salt, pickles or crisps): 477 calories (23.7% from fat), 12.6 g fat (2.3 g saturated fat), 30 g protein, 56.8 g carbohydrate, 63 mg cholesterol, 1,727 mg sodium.

saltsense: By substituting no-salt-added bread, you'll reduce the sodium to 1,322 mg per sandwich. Omitting the bacon reduces it to 602 mg per sandwich.

 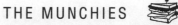

pizza in a flash

makes 4 servings, 2 slices each

I've been making pizza since I was 15 years old. But as my life got busier and leaner, I switched to a prebaked crust. Slather on some fat-free sauce, add some vegetables and low-fat mozzarella cheese, and my pizza is in and out of the oven in 12 minutes. Now that's fast food.

1 12-inch baked pizza crust (such as Boboli)
½ cup fat-free pizza or spaghetti sauce
2 large mushrooms, thinly sliced
½ ounce low-fat turkey pepperoni (about 9 slices)
4 ounces low-fat mozzarella cheese, grated (or 2 ounces grated fat-free mozzarella cheese and 2 ounces grated part-skim mozzarella cheese, mixed together)

½ medium onion, sliced into paper-thin rings and separated
½ red bell pepper, sliced into rings
   Crushed red pepper flakes (optional)

1. Place the oven rack in the lower-middle position and preheat the oven to 450 degrees.

2. Place the crust on a baking sheet. Evenly spread the sauce on the crust to ¼ inch from the edge. Distribute the mushrooms and pepperoni evenly on top of the sauce. Sprinkle on the cheese, then distribute the onion and pepper evenly on top.

3. Bake for 8 to 10 minutes, or until the cheese melts, the onions begin to brown and the crust is crisp. Cut into 8 slices and serve immediately, sprinkling on red pepper flakes at the table, if desired.

 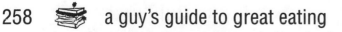

Nutritional information per serving: 389 calories (20.5% from fat), 8.8 g fat (3.6 g saturated fat), 22.1 g protein, 55.7 g carbohydrate, 15 mg cholesterol, 930 mg sodium.

leansuggestions: This pizza can be topped in a variety of ways. Here are a few ideas to get you started:

- Cheeseburger Pizza: Use cooked lean ground beef, substitute reduced-fat extra-sharp cheddar cheese for half of the mozzarella, and use a red onion instead of white.
- New Mexico Pizza: Use fat–free salsa for the sauce, top with 3 ounces shredded grilled chicken breast, 2 tablespoons of canned black beans, rinsed and drained, 2 tablespoons of chopped fresh cilantro and use half grated fat-free mozzarella and half grated reduced-fat cheddar.
- Greek Pizza: Use fat-free spaghetti sauce and top with 2 water-packed artichoke hearts, drained and coarsely chopped, 8 kalamata olives, pitted and chopped, and use half grated mozzarella cheese and half crumbled feta cheese.
- Shrimp Pizza: Use fat-free spaghetti sauce and top with cooked, coarsely chopped shrimp (such as Great Grilled Spicy Shrimp, page 132), top with grated low-fat mozzarella cheese and yellow bell pepper rings.
- North Carolina Pizza: Use the sauce from North Carolina Pulled Turkey Barbecue (page 116), cover with pulled turkey and sprinkle with half grated fat-free mozzarella and half grated reduced-fat cheddar. Top with red onion.

saltsense: About 65 percent of the sodium comes from the crust. If you are on a sodium-restricted food plan, find a crust lower in sodium.

big finish
desserts

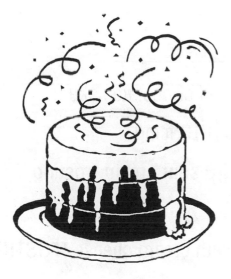

fresh blueberry cobbler

giant black-bottom brownies

double chocolate chip fudge brownies

half-the-fat chocolate chip cookies

oatmeal chocolate chip cookies

chewy brownie cookies

chocolate puddin' cake

deluxe new-fashioned chocolate cake

fat-free fluffy white icing

chocolate fudge sour cream frosting

dark chocolate cake

zucchini fudge cake with cream cheese frosting

peanut butter cake

food processor chocolate frosting

frozen peanut butter pie

velvety chocolate sauce

livin'-large pecan pie

lean n' delicious pumpkin pie

After I lost weight, I knew I couldn't give up

dessert. I spent years testing and endured dozens of failures to create exceptional desserts, especially chocolate ones, that are virtually indistinguishable from the originals.

Double Chocolate Chip Fudge Brownies have the same crisp top and moist, chocolaty interior of ordinary brownies, and they're packed with bits of semisweet chocolate. But a big square contains just 2 grams of fat. For an even bigger thrill, end a special dinner with a slab of Dark Chocolate Cake with Chocolate Sour Cream Fudge Frosting, with only 9 grams of fat per serving, a mere quarter of the fat in the usual kind. In this chapter, you'll find many other desserts you were certain could never be part of a healthful meal plan, like pecan pie and chocolate chip cookies.

Cake made with applesauce drained in a wire-mesh strainer has the moist, tender texture usually achieved with butter. It's made with cocoa powder, which has only 3 fat grams per ounce, whereas 1 ounce of unsweetened chocolate has 16. For the most tender results, I've learned that you must not overmix the batter when incorporating the dry ingredients.

From Fresh Blueberry Cobbler to Frozen Peanut Butter Pie, these desserts have big flavor and big portions—no tiny pans that supposedly serve 60 people. My secret to cutting fat and calories isn't mathematical chicanery but a little kitchen wizardry and a lot of testing.

fresh blueberry cobbler

makes 6 servings

Every summer when I was growing up, my grandmother made fresh blueberry cobbler. The blueberries were plump little gems, and the memory of the fragrance of butter and blueberries drifting from her kitchen still makes my mouth water. Grandmother would wait until her cobbler was just warm and then serve it with vanilla ice cream. I reduced the butter in her original and serve my cobbler with a scoop of low-fat vanilla ice cream.

3 tablespoons unsalted butter

¾ cup all-purpose flour

¾ cup plus 1 tablespoon granulated sugar, *divided*

1 teaspoon baking powder

¼ teaspoon salt

¾ cup 1% milk, at room temperature

2 cups fresh blueberries, picked over, rinsed under cold water and drained well

1. Place the oven rack in the lower-middle position and preheat the oven to 350 degrees. Place the butter in a 9-inch round cake pan and place the pan in the oven to melt, about 3 minutes. (Keep an eye on it so the butter doesn't brown.)

2. In a medium mixing bowl, whisk together the flour, ¾ cup of the sugar, baking powder and salt. Add the milk and whisk until the dry ingredients are just moistened.

3. Pour the batter into the cake pan with the butter; do not stir. Distribute the blueberries over the batter. Sprinkle with the remaining 1 tablespoon sugar. Bake for 40 to 50 minutes, or until golden brown.

Nutritional information per serving: 245 calories (23.7% from fat), 6.5 g fat (3.7 g saturated fat), 2.8 g protein, 46.4 g carbohydrate, 16.8 mg cholesterol, 170 mg sodium.

giant black-bottom brownies

makes 24 brownies

These giant brownies have a chocolate-chip-flecked layer of cheesecake swirled into the dark chocolate batter; thereby combining the best of both brownies and cheesecake.

1½ cups unsweetened applesauce

cream cheese filling
- 2 8-ounce packages nonfat cream cheese, at room temperature
- 1 large egg
- 2 large egg whites
- 1 teaspoon vanilla extract
- 6 tablespoons mini-morsel semisweet chocolate chips

brownie batter
- 2 cups all-purpose flour
- 1⅓ cups unsweetened cocoa powder
- ½ teaspoon salt
- 2 large eggs
- 4 large egg whites
- 2 teaspoons vanilla extract
- 4 cups granulated sugar

1. Place a strainer over a bowl deep enough so the bottom of the strainer doesn't touch the bottom of the bowl. Put the applesauce in the strainer and set aside to drain for 15 minutes; you should have 1 cup drained applesauce.

2. Place the oven rack in the lower-middle position and preheat the oven to 350 degrees. Lightly spray a 13-by-9-inch baking pan with butter-flavored vegetable oil and set aside.

3. To make the filling: Mix the cream cheese, egg, egg whites and vanilla in a large bowl with an electric mixer on medium until combined. Stir in the chocolate chips by hand. Set aside.

4. **To make the batter:** In a medium bowl, whisk together the flour, cocoa powder and salt. Set aside. Place the eggs and egg whites in a large mixing bowl and whisk until foamy. Add the sugar, drained applesauce and vanilla and stir until the sugar has dissolved. Fold in the flour mixture until the dry ingredients are just moistened.

5. Pour half of the brownie batter into the baking pan. Spoon the cream cheese mixture on top. Pour the remaining brownie batter on top of the cream cheese mixture. With a butter knife, make swirls through the batter to produce a marbled effect. Bake for 55 minutes, or until the center is set. Cool on a rack, cut into 2-inch squares and serve.

Nutritional information per brownie: 224 calories (9.7% from fat), 2.4 g fat (1.2 g saturated fat), 6.5 g protein, 47.3 g carbohydrate, 29 mg cholesterol, 158 mg sodium.

double chocolate chip fudge brownies

makes 15 brownies

Everyone who has tasted these brownies mistakes them for their high-fat cousins. Eliminating a stick of butter and substituting drained applesauce blew away almost 800 calories and 93 fat grams. Then I added 2 ounces of chocolate chips, since the addition raised the fat content of each brownie by just a little more than 1 gram. Each big brownie has only 167 calories. What the heck, have a second one!

¾ cup unsweetened applesauce

1 cup all-purpose flour

⅔ cup unsweetened cocoa powder

½ teaspoon salt

1 large egg

2 large egg whites

2 cups granulated sugar

1 teaspoon vanilla extract

¼ cup mini-morsel semisweet
      chocolate chips

1. Place a strainer over a bowl deep enough so the bottom of the strainer doesn't touch the bottom of the bowl. Put the applesauce in the strainer and set aside to drain for 15 minutes; you should have ½ cup drained applesauce.

2. Place the oven rack in the center and preheat the oven to 350 degrees. Lightly spray an 11-by-7-by-1½-inch baking pan with the butter-flavored vegetable oil.

3. In a medium bowl, whisk together the flour, cocoa and salt.

4. In a large mixing bowl, whisk together the egg and egg whites until bubbly. Add the sugar, drained applesauce and vanilla and stir until the sugar has dissolved. Stir in the flour mixture and chocolate chips until the dry ingredients are just moistened.

5. Pour the batter into the prepared pan and bake for 30 minutes for a fudgy center, 35 minutes for a cakey center. Cool on a rack, cut into fifteen 2-inch squares and serve.

Nutritional information per brownie: 167 calories (11.1% from fat), 2 g fat (1.1 g saturated fat), 2.6 g protein, 38.2 g carbohydrate, 14 mg cholesterol, 84 mg sodium.

cookingtip: To make these brownies even more decadent, use ½ cup chocolate chips. This will increase the calories per serving to 185 and the fat to 3.2 grams.

half-the-fat chocolate chip cookies

makes 40 cookies

Chocolate chip cookies made from the original Tollhouse recipe used to be my favorite. I cut out half the fat and left all the terrific flavor.

¾ cup unsweetened applesauce
2½ cups all-purpose flour
1 teaspoon baking soda
½ teaspoon salt
½ cup soft tub margarine, at room temperature
¾ cup granulated sugar

¾ cup light brown sugar
1 large egg
1 large egg white
1 teaspoon vanilla extract
1 12-ounce bag Hershey's reduced-fat chocolate chips
½ cup coarsely chopped pecans

1. Place a strainer over a bowl deep enough so the bottom of the strainer doesn't touch the bottom of the bowl. Put the applesauce in the strainer and set aside to drain for 15 minutes; you should have ½ cup drained applesauce.

2. Place the oven rack in the lower-middle position and preheat the oven to 375 degrees.

3. In a medium mixing bowl, whisk together the flour, baking soda and salt and set aside.

4. Put the margarine in a large bowl and mix with an electric mixer on medium-high for 2 minutes, until light. Add the applesauce and mix on medium-high until light. Add the sugar and brown sugar and mix for 3 minutes on medium-high until fluffy. Add the egg and egg white, one at a time, mixing for 30 seconds after each addition. Add the vanilla and mix for 15 seconds. Fold in the flour mixture by hand and then the chocolate chips and pecans; do not overmix.

 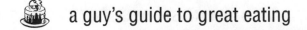

5. Drop the dough by heaping tablespoons onto ungreased baking sheets. Bake for 14 minutes, or until light brown. Remove from the pans and cool on wire racks.

Nutritional information per cookie: 118 calories (32.8% from fat), 4.3 g fat (1.6 g saturated fat), 1.1 g protein, 12.9 g carbohydrate, 5.3 mg cholesterol, 70 mg sodium.

leansuggestion: To trim the fat even further, omit the pecans. Each cookie will have 108 calories (27.5% from fat) and 3.3 fat grams.

oatmeal chocolate chip cookies

makes about 40 cookies

Doug Bunn, a listener on a Raleigh radio program, heard me say that nonfat plain yogurt makes a terrific substitute for vegetable oil in cookie recipes. After the show, he put together a batch using a ratio of one-third canola oil to two-thirds nonfat plain yogurt. Success! The cookies were chewy but not sticky, and he'd cut almost 110 fat grams. Doug told me that preparing them "requires the assistance of an eight-year-old for quality assurance."

¾ cup all-purpose flour
¾ cup whole wheat flour
½ teaspoon baking soda
½ teaspoon salt
½ cup plain nonfat yogurt
¼ cup canola oil
1 cup light brown sugar

½ cup granulated sugar
1 large egg
1 teaspoon vanilla extract
3 cups uncooked quick oatmeal
   (not instant or old-fashioned)
1 12-ounce bag Hershey's reduced-
   fat chocolate chips

1. Place the oven rack in the lower-middle position and preheat the oven to 375 degrees.

2. In a medium mixing bowl, whisk together the flour, whole wheat flour, baking soda and salt.

3. In a large mixing bowl, beat the yogurt and oil with an electric mixer on medium-high for 3 minutes, or until emulsified. Add the brown sugar and sugar and mix for 4 minutes, or until creamy. Add the egg and vanilla and mix for 30 seconds. Scrape down the sides of the bowl. Add the oatmeal and mix on medium for 30 seconds, until combined. Add the flour mixture and mix on low until just moistened. Stir in the chocolate chips by hand.

 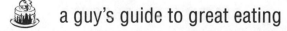

4.   Drop the dough by rounded tablespoons onto ungreased cookie sheets (I use an insu-
lated cookie sheet) and bake for 13 to 14 minutes, or until the tops are golden brown.

Nutritional information per cookie: 111 calories (25.5% from fat), 3.1 g fat (1.4 g saturated fat),
2 g protein, 20.1 g carbohydrate, 5 mg cholesterol, 42 mg sodium.

cookingtip: Greasing the cookie sheet causes the cookies to spread too much. Use a thin
metal spatula to remove them from the sheet.

 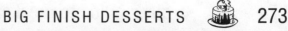

chewy brownie cookies

makes about 36 cookies

When I sampled the original version of these cookies, I could not believe how chewy and delicious they were. When I learned that they contained two-thirds of a cup of shortening, I knew why. I loved their flavor and chewiness, but I had to make them lower in fat and calories.

I halved the shortening and added drained applesauce to blow away 580 calories and 65 fat grams. Using reduced-fat chocolate chips slashed the fat even more. These cookies are just as chewy and chocolaty as the original but have half the fat.

⅔ cup unsweetened applesauce
⅓ cup butter-flavored vegetable shortening
1½ cups packed light brown sugar
1½ cups all-purpose flour
⅓ cup unsweetened cocoa powder
½ teaspoon salt

¼ teaspoon baking soda
1 teaspoon vanilla extract
1 large egg
1 large egg white
1 12-ounce bag Hershey's reduced-fat chocolate chips

1. Place a strainer over a bowl deep enough so the bottom of the strainer doesn't touch the bottom of the bowl. Put the applesauce in the strainer and set aside to drain for 15 minutes; you should have ⅓ cup drained applesauce.

2. Meanwhile, place the oven rack in the center and preheat the oven to 375 degrees.

3. In a large bowl, beat the shortening for 2 minutes with an electric mixer on medium-high. Scrape down the sides of the bowl, add the brown sugar and beat together for 4 minutes, or until fluffy.

 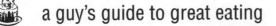

4.   Whisk together the flour, cocoa, salt and baking soda in a medium mixing bowl.

5.   Add the drained applesauce and vanilla to the shortening mixture and mix on medium-high for 1 minute. Add the egg and egg white and mix for 20 seconds. Scrape down the sides of the bowl, add the flour mixture and beat on low until just moistened. Stir in the chocolate chips by hand.

6.   Drop the dough by rounded tablespoons onto ungreased baking sheets, 2 inches apart. Bake for 10 to 11 minutes, or until the cookies are set. Cool for 2 minutes on the baking sheet. Place the cookies on wire racks to cool completely.

Nutritional information per cookie: 100 calories (29.8% from fat), 3.3 g fat (1.8 g saturated fat), 1.1 g protein, 17 g carbohydrate, 6 mg cholesterol, 41 mg sodium.

chocolate puddin' cake

makes 6 servings

This is an easy cake, and it contains only 1 fat gram per serving. Before it is baked, the top looks like a mud puddle. Don't worry. Almost magically, a fudgy pudding appears on the bottom. The cake itself is like a brownie. I serve it with a scoop of low-fat vanilla ice cream and drizzle some of the warm sauce over all.

½ cup unsweetened applesauce

pudding
½ cup granulated sugar
½ cup packed dark brown sugar
¼ cup unsweetened cocoa powder

cake batter
1 cup all-purpose flour
¾ cups granulated sugar
3 tablespoons unsweetened cocoa powder
2 teaspoons baking powder
¼ teaspoon salt
½ cup skim milk
1½ teaspoons vanilla extract

1. Place a strainer over a bowl deep enough so the bottom of the strainer doesn't touch the bottom of the bowl. Put the applesauce in the strainer and set aside to drain for 15 minutes; you should have ⅓ cup drained applesauce.

2. Place the oven rack in the lower-middle position and preheat the oven to 350 degrees.

3. **To make the pudding:** Whisk together the sugar, brown sugar and cocoa in a medium mixing bowl and set aside.

4. **To make the cake batter:** In a medium mixing bowl, whisk together the flour, sugar, cocoa, baking powder and salt. Add the milk, drained applesauce and vanilla and whisk until smooth.

5. Pour the cake batter into an ungreased 8-by-8-by-2-inch baking pan. Spread the pudding mixture over evenly; do not mix it in. Pour 1 cup hot water evenly over the top of the pudding mixture; do not mix in. Bake for 35 to 40 minutes, or until the center is almost set.

6. Transfer the baking pan to a wire rack and cool for 15 minutes. Serve immediately.

Nutritional information per serving: 306 calories (3.1% from fat), 1.1 g fat (0.5 g saturated fat), 3.8 g protein, 75.6 g carbohydrate, trace of cholesterol, 227 mg sodium.

cooking**tip**: This dessert does not keep well. Discard any leftovers.

 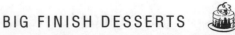

deluxe new-fashioned chocolate cake

makes 15 servings

Deluxe old-fashioned chocolate cake made from the recipe on the back of the baking chocolate box contains 214 fat grams. By replacing most of the chocolate with cocoa powder, cutting
back on the eggs and making a few more alterations, I eliminated 124 fat grams and more
than 1,000 calories. Frost with Fat-Free Fluffy White Icing (page 280) or Chocolate Fudge
Sour Cream Frosting (page 281).

¾ cup unsweetened applesauce
½ cup unsweetened cocoa powder
1 ounce baking chocolate, broken
   into pieces
2¼ cups cake flour
1 teaspoon baking powder
1 teaspoon baking soda
½ teaspoon salt

¼ cup unsalted butter, at room
   temperature
1⅔ cups packed light brown sugar
1 teaspoon vanilla extract
1 large egg yolk, at room
   temperature
3 large eggs, at room temperature

1. Place a strainer over a bowl deep enough so the bottom of the strainer doesn't touch
the bottom of the bowl. Put the applesauce in the strainer and set aside to drain for
15 minutes; you should have ½ cup drained applesauce.

2. Place the cocoa, ⅓ cup water and baking chocolate in a small heavy-bottomed
saucepan. Over low heat, stir constantly until the chocolate melts. Remove from the
heat and cool.

3. Place the oven rack in the center and preheat the oven to 350 degrees. Lightly spray a
13-by-9-inch baking pan with a vegetable-oil-and-flour spray such as Baker's Joy.

4. Sift the cake flour, baking powder, baking soda and salt together three times.

5. In a large bowl, cream the butter for 2 minutes with an electric mixer on medium-high, until light. Beat in the brown sugar and mix for 3 minutes, or until fluffy. Add the drained applesauce and vanilla and beat for 1 minute. Add the cooled chocolate mixture and mix for 1 minute. Add the egg yolk and mix for 20 seconds. Add the eggs, one at a time, mixing for 20 seconds each. Add the sifted flour mixture and mix on low until just blended. Add ½ cup water and mix until just incorporated.

6. Scrape the sides of the bowl and stir the batter a few times. Pour the batter into the prepared pan, smoothing the surface, and bake for 35 minutes, or until a toothpick inserted into the center comes out clean. Cool on a rack. Cut into 2½-by-3-inch rectangles and serve.

Nutritional information per serving (unfrosted): 186 calories (29% from fat), 6 g fat (3.2 g saturated fat), 3.3 g protein, 31.6 g carbohydrate, 65 mg cholesterol, 180 mg sodium.

fat-free fluffy white icing

makes about 2 cups, enough to frost a 13-by-9-inch cake.

This icing tops a chocolate cake in a special, fat-free way. The sugar syrup is hot enough to cook the egg whites.

1 cup granulated sugar
¼ teaspoon cream of tartar
Pinch of salt

2 large egg whites
1 teaspoon vanilla extract

1. Combine ½ cup water, the sugar, cream of tartar and salt in a small heavy-bottomed saucepan and bring to a boil, stirring to dissolve the sugar. Boil, without stirring, for 5 minutes.

2. Meanwhile, in a large bowl, beat the egg whites until frothy with an electric mixer on high. With the mixer running, slowly pour the hot syrup over the egg whites. Continue beating until it forms stiff, glossy peaks. Beat in the vanilla. Spread the icing on the cake.

Nutritional information per ¹⁄₁₅ serving of a 13-by-9-inch cake: 53 calories (0% from fat), 0 g fat (0 g saturated fat), 0.5 g protein, 13.4 g carbohydrate, 0 mg cholesterol, 25 mg sodium.

chocolate fudge sour cream frosting

makes 2½ cups, enough to fill and frost a 9-inch two-layer cake or a 13-by-9-inch cake

When I was a kid, one of my favorite things to do was lick the mixer bowl and beaters when my mom made chocolate buttercream frosting. This is an updated version of my favorite frosting, minus most of the fat and many of the calories. When you make it, watch out for bowl-lickers sneaking up behind you.

5 tablespoons semisweet chocolate chips
½ cup low-fat margarine (2 fat grams per tablespoon), at room temperature
3 tablespoons reduced-fat sour cream
4 teaspoons vanilla extract

¾ cup Dutch-process cocoa powder (such as Hershey's European-style or Droste), sifted
1 pound confectioners' sugar, sifted, *divided*

1. Melt the chocolate chips in the top of a double boiler.

2. Beat the margarine, sour cream and vanilla in a small mixing bowl with an electric mixer on low until combined. Add the melted chocolate and beat on low until smooth. Add the cocoa powder and beat on low until combined.

3. Add half the confectioners' sugar and beat on low until it disappears, about 30 seconds. Add the remaining confectioners' sugar and beat on low until smooth and spreadable, about 30 seconds. Spread the frosting on the cake.

Nutritional information per tablespoon: 62 calories (17% from fat), 1.2 g fat (0.4 g saturated fat), 0.4 g protein, 13.6 g carbohydrate, 0.6 mg cholesterol, 23 mg sodium.

cookingtips: If the frosting is too thick, mix in 1 to 2 teaspoons water.
- If you are unable to locate Dutch-process cocoa powder, substitute regular cocoa.

dark chocolate cake

makes 15 servings

When my wife and I lived in Illinois, we had a wonderful neighbor who presented us with an outstanding hot-water chocolate cake one Christmas. The cake had a deep, rich color and an equally intense chocolate flavor.

My version tastes so good, you won't believe that it has only 206 calories and 4.5 fat grams. Like the original, it has a dense texture and a brawny chocolate flavor. If you like, frost it with Fat-Free Fluffy White Icing (page 280), or dust it with confectioners' sugar.

½ cup unsweetened applesauce

1¾ cups all-purpose flour

¾ cup unsweetened cocoa powder

2 teaspoons baking powder

1 teaspoon salt

¼ teaspoon baking soda

4 tablespoons unsalted butter, at room temperature

2 cups granulated sugar

2 large eggs, at room temperature

¾ cup skim milk, at room temperature

2 teaspoons vanilla extract

1. Place a strainer over a bowl deep enough so the bottom of the strainer doesn't touch the bottom of the bowl. Put the applesauce in the strainer and set aside to drain for 15 minutes; you should have ¼ cup drained applesauce.

2. Place the oven rack in the lower-middle position and preheat the oven to 350 degrees. Spray a 13-by-9-by-2-inch baking pan with a vegetable-oil-and-flour spray, such as Baker's Joy.

3. In a medium bowl, whisk together the flour, cocoa, baking powder, salt and baking soda and set aside.

4. Place the drained applesauce and butter in a large mixing bowl. Beat with an electric mixer on medium-high for 3 minutes. Scrape down the sides of the bowl, add the sugar and beat for 3 minutes, or until creamy. With the mixer running, add the eggs, one at a time, and mix for 25 seconds each. Add the milk and vanilla and mix on medium for 20 seconds, or until incorporated. Scrape down the sides of the bowl, add the flour mixture and beat on low until just moistened.

5. Add ⅔ cup boiling water to the batter. Mix on low until just incorporated; the batter will be thin.

6. Scrape the sides of the bowl and stir the batter a few times. Pour the batter into the prepared pan and bake for 35 minutes, or until a toothpick inserted in the center comes out clean. Cool completely on a wire rack for 1½ hours. Serve.

Nutritional information per unfrosted serving: 206 calories (19.7% from fat), 4.5 g fat (2.5 g saturated fat), 3.4 g protein, 41.2 g carbohydrate, 37 mg cholesterol, 219 mg sodium.

zucchini fudge cake with cream cheese frosting

makes 16 servings

Ground cinnamon lends a Mexican note to this dense cake, and buttermilk adds rich, tangy flavor. The zucchini makes the cake unbelievably moist.

1¼ cups unsweetened applesauce
2 cups grated zucchini
2½ cups all-purpose flour
4 tablespoons cocoa powder
2 teaspoons ground cinnamon
1½ teaspoons baking powder
½ teaspoon salt
¼ teaspoon baking soda
¼ cup unsalted butter, at room temperature
1¼ cups granulated sugar
1 large egg

1 large egg white
1 teaspoon vanilla extract
½ cup low-fat buttermilk
¼ cup mini-morsel semisweet chocolate chips

frosting
1½ cups confectioners' sugar
4 ounces Neufchâtel cheese, at room temperature
½ teaspoon vanilla extract

1. Place a strainer over a bowl deep enough so the bottom of the strainer doesn't touch the bottom of the bowl. Put the applesauce in the strainer and set aside to drain for 15 minutes; you should have ¾ cup drained applesauce.

2. Place the grated zucchini in the center of a heavy-duty paper towel, gather up the corners and twist over the sink until liquid no longer drips from the zucchini. Set aside.

3. Place the oven rack in the lower-middle position and preheat the oven to 350 degrees. Spray a 13-by-9-by-2-inch baking pan with a vegetable-oil-and-flour spray, such as Baker's Joy.

4. In a medium mixing bowl, whisk together the flour, cocoa powder, cinnamon, baking powder, salt and baking soda. Set aside.

5. Place the drained applesauce and butter in a large mixing bowl and mix with an electric mixer on medium-high for 4 minutes, or until light. Scrape down the sides of the bowl, add the sugar and mix on medium-high for 4 minutes, until light and fluffy. Beat in the egg and mix for 25 seconds. Beat in the egg white and vanilla and mix for 25 seconds, or until incorporated. Beat in the buttermilk on medium for 20 seconds, or until incorporated; the batter will appear curdled.

6. Add the zucchini and mix on medium-low for 20 seconds, or until combined. Add the flour mixture and chocolate chips and mix on low until just moistened, about 15 seconds.

7. Scrape the sides of the bowl and stir the batter a few times. Pour the batter into the prepared pan, smoothing the top. Bake for 40 minutes, or until a toothpick inserted in the center comes out clean. Place the pan on a wire rack and let cool completely, about 2 hours.

8. **To make the frosting:** Place the confectioners' sugar, Neufchâtel cheese and vanilla in a food processor with the steel blade in place. Process, pulsing, for 5 to 7 seconds, or until smooth. Spread the frosting on the cooled cake. Cut the cake into 2-by-3-inch pieces and serve.

Nutritional information per serving: 266 calories (21.4% from fat), 6.3 g fat (3.7 g saturated fat), 3.8 g protein, 51.1 g carbohydrate, 26 mg cholesterol, 151 mg sodium.

peanut butter cake

makes 24 servings

When my friend Peter recently had a birthday, I created a peanut butter cake using reduced-fat peanut butter and frosted it with low-fat chocolate frosting. It had less than 3 grams of fat per serving, and Peter said it was his best birthday cake ever.

½ cup unsweetened applesauce
2 cups sifted cake flour
3 teaspoons baking powder
½ cup reduced-fat peanut butter
1 cup light brown sugar

1 teaspoon vanilla extract
2 large eggs
1 large egg white
¾ cup skim milk

1. Place a strainer over a bowl deep enough so the bottom of the strainer doesn't touch the bottom of the bowl. Put the applesauce in the strainer and set aside to drain for 15 minutes; you should have ⅓ cup drained applesauce.

2. Place the oven rack in the lower-middle position and preheat the oven to 350 degrees. Spray a 13-by-9-by-2-inch baking pan with a vegetable-oil-and-flour spray, such as Baker's Joy.

3. Whisk together the sifted cake flour and baking powder in a medium mixing bowl. Set aside.

4. In a large bowl, beat the peanut butter with an electric mixer on medium for 2 minutes, or until light. Scrape down the sides of the bowl, add the drained applesauce and mix on medium-high for 2 minutes, or until incorporated. Scrape down the sides of the bowl and beat in the brown sugar for 3 minutes, or until creamy. Beat in the

 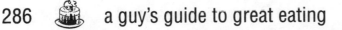

vanilla. Beat in the eggs, one at a time, mixing for 25 seconds each. Beat in the egg white for 25 seconds. Beat in the milk until incorporated, about 20 seconds. Add the flour mixture and mix on low until moistened, about 15 seconds.

5. Scrape the sides of the bowl and stir the batter a few times. Pour the batter into the prepared pan and bake for 20 to 25 minutes, or until the center of the cake springs back when pressed. Cool completely in the pan on a wire rack. Cut into 2-inch squares and serve.

Nutritional information per serving (unfrosted): 94 calories (22% from fat), 2.3 g fat (0.5 g saturated fat), 2.7 g protein, 15.9 g carbohydrate, 9 mg cholesterol, 98 mg sodium.

Nutritional information per frosted serving: 160 calories (16.6% from fat), 2.9 g fat (0.5 g saturated fat), 3 g protein, 31.6 g carbohydrate, 9 mg cholesterol, 125 mg sodium.

lean suggestion: When the cake is completely cooled, frost it with Food Processor Chocolate Frosting (page 288).

food processor chocolate frosting

makes about 1½ cups, enough to frost a 13-by-9-inch cake

This frosting is smooth and dark and rich. If you didn't know better, you'd think it was high in fat.

2⅔ cups confectioners' sugar, sifted, *divided*

6 tablespoons low-fat margarine (2 fat grams per tablespoon)

½ cup Dutch-process cocoa powder (such as Hershey's European-style or Droste)

1 teaspoon vanilla extract

2–3 teaspoons skim milk

Place half of the sifted sugar, the margarine, cocoa and vanilla in the bowl of a food processor with the steel blade in place. Process, pulsing, for 5 to 7 seconds, or until the sugar dissolves. Add the remaining sugar and 2 teaspoons of the milk and process, pulsing, for 5 to 7 seconds, or until smooth. If the frosting is too thick, add 1 more teaspoon of milk and process until combined. Spread the frosting on the cake.

Nutritional information per tablespoon: 66 calories (9% from fat), 0.7 g fat (trace of saturated fat), 0.3 g protein, 15.7 g carbohydrate, trace of cholesterol, 27 mg sodium.

cookingtip: If you can't find Dutch-process cocoa powder, substitute an equal amount of regular cocoa powder.

frozen peanut butter pie

makes 8 servings

My next door neighbor Julie makes this terrific peanut butter pie for her husband, Rob. It seems decadent, with 397 calories and 12 fat grams per slice, until you learn that the original delivered 618 calories and 40 fat grams per slice.

1 large egg white
1 store-bought reduced-fat graham cracker pie crust
1 8-ounce package Healthy Choice fat-free cream cheese, at room temperature
¾ cup reduced-fat peanut butter

1 cup confectioners' sugar
⅓ cup skim milk
8 ounces fat-free whipped topping, thawed
Chocolate syrup, such as Velvety Chocolate Sauce (page 290)
1 tablespoon chopped peanuts

1. Place the oven rack in the center and preheat the oven to 375 degrees.

2. In a small bowl, whisk the egg white until bubbly. Brush the pie crust with the beaten egg white. Bake for 5 minutes. Cool on a wire rack for 15 minutes.

3. Meanwhile, in a large bowl, beat the cream cheese and peanut butter with an electric mixer on low until smooth. Add the confectioners' sugar and milk and mix until combined. With a rubber spatula, fold in the whipped topping. Spoon the filling into the prepared pie crust and freeze for 8 hours.

4. Before cutting, drizzle a little chocolate syrup over the top of the pie and sprinkle with the peanuts.

Nutritional information per serving: 397 calories (27.5% from fat), 12 g fat (2.5 g saturated fat), 14.3 g protein, 51.7 g carbohydrate, 5 mg cholesterol, 408 mg sodium.

velvety chocolate sauce

makes about 2 cups

Ever since I was a child, I've loved chocolate sauce on my ice cream. This fresh chocolate sauce is better than any I've ever bought.

- 1 cup granulated sugar
- ½ cup Dutch-process unsweetened cocoa powder (such as Hershey's European-style or Droste)
- 2 tablespoons all-purpose flour
- ½ teaspoon salt
- 1 tablespoon unsalted butter
- 1 teaspoon vanilla extract

Over hot water in a double boiler, stir together the sugar, cocoa powder, flour and salt. Gradually stir in 1 cup boiling water. Cook, stirring constantly, until slightly thickened and smooth, 5 to 7 minutes. Remove from the heat, stir in the butter and vanilla and cool. Cover and refrigerate for 2 hours before serving. This sauce keeps, refrigerated, for 2 weeks.

Nutritional information per tablespoon: 31 calories (14.3% from fat), 0.5 g fat (0.2 g saturated fat), 0.3 g protein, 7.3 g carbohydrate, 0.9 mg cholesterol, 34 mg sodium.

cookingtip: If you are unable to locate Dutch-process unsweetened cocoa powder, substitute regular unsweetened.

saltsense: If you are on a sodium-restricted food plan, omit the salt.

 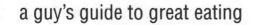

livin'-large pecan pie

makes 8 servings

Although this pie has half the fat of a regular pecan pie, its flavor is virtually indistinguishable from the original.

2 large egg yolks
1½ tablespoons unsalted butter, melted
6 large egg whites
1⅓ cups dark corn syrup
1⅓ cups granulated sugar
1¼ teaspoons vanilla extract

¾ cup pecan halves, sliced lengthwise into slivers
1 9-inch unbaked store-bought reduced-fat deep-dish pie crust

1. Place the oven rack in the lower-middle position and preheat the oven to 350 degrees.

2. In a large mixing bowl, whisk together the egg yolks and melted butter until combined. Add the egg whites and whisk until frothy. Whisk in the corn syrup, sugar and vanilla until the sugar has dissolved. Stir in the pecans.

3. Pour the mixture into the pie crust, place the pie pan on a jelly-roll pan, and bake for 60 to 65 minutes, or until a knife inserted halfway between the center and the edge comes out clean. Cool on a wire rack and serve.

Nutritional information per serving: 508 calories (23.5% from fat), 13.3 g fat (3.3 g saturated fat), 5.3 g protein, 93.7 g carbohydrate, 59 mg cholesterol, 383 mg sodium.

leansuggestion: A small scoop of low-fat vanilla ice cream is wonderful on this pie.

 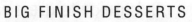

lean n' delicious pumpkin pie

makes 8 servings

Everyone loves a slice of warm pumpkin pie as the perfect ending to a Thanksgiving meal. You can indulge and feel no guilt at all.

1 large egg
2 large egg whites
1 15-ounce can solid pack pumpkin
1 12-ounce can evaporated skim milk
¾ cup granulated sugar
½ teaspoon salt

1 teaspoon ground cinnamon
½ teaspoon ground ginger
¼ teaspoon ground cloves
   Pinch of fresh-grated nutmeg
1 9-inch unbaked reduced-fat pie
   crust (3 fat grams per serving)

1. Place the oven rack in the center and preheat the oven to 425 degrees.

2. Whisk the egg and egg whites in a large mixing bowl until frothy. Whisk in the pumpkin and evaporated milk until combined. Whisk in the sugar, salt, cinnamon, ginger, cloves and nutmeg and whisk until the sugar has dissolved.

3. Pour the filling into the pie crust and bake for 15 minutes. Reduce the oven temperature to 350 degrees and bake for 20 to 30 minutes more, or until a toothpick inserted into the center comes out clean. Remove from the oven and cool to room temperature on a wire rack. Serve.

Nutritional information per serving: 217 calories (16.2% from fat), 3.9 g fat (0.9 g saturated fat), 7.9 g protein, 39.7 g carbohydrate, 28.5 mg cholesterol, 227 mg sodium.

leansuggestions: Serve with fat-free, nondairy whipped topping.
  ♦ ¾ cup Sugar Twin sugar substitute (spoonable) may be substituted for the sugar.

 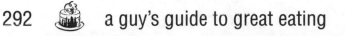

guy talk

indispensable kitchen tools

cheese grater—Hard cheeses, such as Parmesan and Romano, deliver infinitely more flavor when freshly grated.

garlic press—A garlic press saves tons of time. Buy a forged metal garlic press, since the plastic ones don't work well and break quickly.

instant-read thermometer—The best of the best is Owen Instruments Thermapen 5 (which can be purchased from *The Baker's Catalogue:* 1 (800) 827-6836). The Polder Cooking Thermometer/Timer is reasonably priced and is also available from *The Baker's Catalogue.*

knife sharpener—The most dangerous tool in a kitchen is a dull knife. A Chef's Choice knife sharpener keeps knives keen.

knives—Good knives aren't cheap, and they shouldn't be. A quality knife is a lifetime investment. Check out the knife section of any good cookware store. Catalogs may offer better prices, but you don't have the chance to test-drive the knife. I recommend J. A. Henckels Four Star and Wüsthof-Trident brands.

oven thermometer—Buy the best one you can find and have your oven adjusted if necessary.

pepper mill—I own two, one for black peppercorns and one for white. The Unicorn Magnum Plus Restaurant Use Peppermill is easy to fill and has a great range of grinds.

salad spinner—Not just for drying lettuce, but also for cilantro, parsley, cabbage and spinach.

scale—A digital scale is ideal for accurate weighing. They cost between $40 and $60. If you don't want to spend that much, buy a postal scale. You'll soon find it indispensable.

when you hit the road

Restaurateurs count dollars, not calories or fat grams. Fortunately for them, they're not with us when we step on the scale at the end of the week. When you dine out, keep in mind these strategies:

- Half an hour before leaving the house, have a small, nutritious snack. A bowl of soup loaded with vegetables and a little pasta or rice works wonders for me. Fresh vegetables dipped in low-fat or fat-free salad dressing will also take the edge off your hunger.
- In Italian restaurants, order broiled fish drizzled with a little meatless marinara sauce.
- In Greek restaurants, consider broiled lean lamb with steamed vegetables. Tell them to hold the sauce.
- In pizza houses, avoid the meats and load the pizza with vegetables. Most pizza places will be happy to use less cheese on top.
- In Chinese restaurants, tell the waitperson that you'd like the chef to stir-fry with only a small amount of oil. Or order a steamed vegetable dish and mix it with a stir-fried dish to cut the fat content in half.
- Wherever you dine out, steer clear of cheese (9 fat grams per ounce), cream sauces (10.5 fat grams per 2 tablespoons), sausage (80 percent of calories from fat), mayonnaise (11 fat grams per tablespoon), sour cream (5 fat grams per 2 tablespoons) and butter (11.5 fat grams per tablespoon). Avoid anything fried or sauced.
- Look for steamed vegetables, fresh greens and broiled, grilled or baked meats. Ask for salad dressing on the side, dip your fork in the dressing, then spear a piece of lettuce or a vegetable. Stay away from "all-you-can-eat buffet" meals. Ask for fresh fruit or sorbet for dessert.

 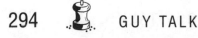

- If your main course is far larger than expected, ask for a doggy bag, put half your meal in it and then eat the remainder.
- Make your waitperson your ally. If the restaurant isn't busy, the chef may be able to prepare something special just for you—if you ask. If your server helped you accomplish your healthful dining goal, please reward him or her.

 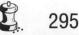

acknowledgments

I am deeply indebted to the following people:

If my wife, Susan, hadn't relinquished the stove to me more than 25 years ago, I wouldn't have taught myself to cook. Susan's ceaseless belief and love have made all things possible for me. I am also grateful to her for testing and tasting recipes to make certain that even a kitchen novice will succeed.

Without Sharon Sanders, who discovered me in 1992 and told all of Chicago about my food, this cookbook would not have been possible.

Anne Fletcher, a wonderful author and an even better friend, deserves a big thank you for her insights and ideas. Anne was right to tell me to stop getting ready to write the proposal for this cookbook and "just do it!"

Bev Mills has shared her wisdom about food writing, and my efforts are better because of her.

My editor, Rux Martin, clarifies my thoughts, supports my ideas and helps me write books that are better than they otherwise would have been.

My publisher, Barry Estabrook, has been enormously supportive. Barry's word is his bond.

My recipes and stories have been greatly strengthened by Jessica Sherman's superior copyediting.

Lori Galvin-Frost at Houghton Mifflin Company is a gem. The many roles she played in bringing this cookbook to fruition are too numerous to list; yet, she made them all seem effortless.

To Tom Mauer, who suggested this cookbook in the first place, I offer my thanks. It would not be as good as it is without his frequent tweaks.

Bob Mauer is my brother in more ways than one. His spiritual journey has brought me universal insights.

Bill Wurch, my attorney and friend, has been very generous with his astute legal opinions and concise personal observations.

Scott Davis is my idea guy. I appreciate his intuition and creativity.

I wish to thank Fred Thompson, Aliza Green and Cris Mata for making my food look so incredible and edible on television.

Thank you to all the talented and dedicated people at UNC-TV (PBS) in North Carolina, not only for allowing me to appear on television, but for making everything I do there look great.

To Renee McCoy, Bill Leslie, Raymond Farrar, Spencer Jenkins and all the great people at WRAL-TV (CBS) in Raleigh, thank you for making it possible for me to appear on television regularly for more than five years.

To all the terrific people at QVC, thank you. You make appearing on national television a wonderful experience each and every time.

To my readers at Chicago's *Daily Herald* and the *Herald-Sun*, you keep me writing.

To Kim Spurr, thank you for bringing my column to the *Durham Herald-Sun* in 1995.

Several guys contributed their recipes to this endeavor: William Barton, Doug Bunn, Al Carson and Tom Mauer. Thank you.

In memoriam: Carole VanGoethem was a very special lady. She wrote me my first fan letter when my cable cooking series began airing in Chicago in 1993. Carole was one of my biggest followers until her untimely passing in 1997.

Index